The International Library of Psychology

ISAAC AND OEDIPUS

Founded by C. K. Ogden

The International Library of Psychology

PSYCHOLOGY AND RELIGION
In 6 Volumes

I	Hindu Psychology	*Akhilananda*
II	Religious Conversion	*de Sanctis*
III	The Psychology of Religious Mysticism	*Leuba*
IV	Indian Psychology	*Sinha*
V	Isaac and Oedipus	*Wellisch*
VI	Man in his Relationships	*Westmann*

ISAAC AND OEDIPUS

A Study in Biblical Psychology of the Sacrifice of Isaac *The Akedah*

E WELLISCH

Routledge
Taylor & Francis Group
LONDON AND NEW YORK

First published in 1954
by Routledge

Reprinted in 1999, 2000, 2001
by Routledge
2 Park Square, Milton Park, Abingdon, Oxon, OX14 4RN

Simultaneously published in the USA and Canada by Routledge
711 Third Avenue, New York, NY 10017

Transferred to Digital Printing 2007

Routledge is an imprint of the Taylor & Francis Group

First issued in paperback 2013

British Library Cataloguing in Publication Data
A CIP catalogue record for this book
is available from the British Library

Isaac and Oedipus

ISBN 978-0-415-21114-7 (hbk)
ISBN 978-0-415-86547-0 (pbk)

TO MY SON

Preface

THIS is a religious-psychological study of the father-son relationship. It represents a re-evaluation of the Oedipus Complex and is based on the exposition of the twenty-second chapter of Genesis, the Sacrifice of Isaac.

The thesis of the study is that phenomena described in the Bible provide a unique contribution to psychological truth. The analysis of the story of the Sacrifice of Isaac shows that it contains mental mechanisms which are characteristic for the Oedipus situation; but it also reveals mental experiences which differ in important aspects from this situation. These experiences are specific for Jewish and Christian religion, or —to use a term which expresses the essential bond between them—for Biblical religion. Mental experiences and mechanisms characteristic of Biblical religion occur in every person and can be observed clinically. This opens possibilities for a new field of psychiatric research.

I am deeply grateful for the encouragement given to me in the course of this study by Dr. Kenneth Cameron, Physician of the Department of Child Psychiatry at the Maudsley and Bethlem Royal Hospitals, London.

I am also very thankful for kind interest and advice from the Rev. Stafford Wright, Principal of Tyndale Hall Theological College, Bristol.

Invaluable criticism and help was given to me by Dr.

R. J. Z. Werblowsky of Leeds University, for which I am very much indebted.

Mr. H. J. Sants of the Crayford Child Guidance Clinic has given me most valuable assistance in the work and in the reading of the manuscript and I thank him most sincerely for this.

Dr. H. Frankfort, Director of the Warburg Institute of the University of London and his staff have generously helped me in my studies of the iconography of the Sacrifice of Isaac and have kindly lent me two photographs for reproduction. For this I wish to express my gratitude. The religious icon is reproduced by kind permission of the British Museum.

I should like to thank the Lord Chamberlain for kindly permitting me to use the official photograph 'The Sacrifice of Isaac' as an illustration.

E. W.

November 1953

Contents

Contents

Illustrations

Introduction

'Honour thy father and thy mother:
That thy days may be long upon the land
Which the Lord thy God giveth thee.'

EXODUS, XX, 12

B

Introduction

PSYCHOLOGY is based on the relationships of parents to children and children to parents. All other human relationships are modifications or extensions of the basic experiences within the family.

The relationships between parents and children undergo a fundamentally important process of development from a morally lower to a morally higher form. This process occurred during the development of the human race and occurs during the development of the individual. It is a phylogenetic and ontogenetic process. On the integration of the filio-parental relationships depends all cultural progress and all such progress is nothing else than a higher moral development of our personal relationships with our parents and children.

Our whole personal life and happiness is profoundly influenced by the way in which we behave towards our parents and children. This decides, in the words of the Decalogue, whether or not the days will be long upon the land which the Lord our God giveth us.

The moral relationships of parents to their children can be considered in three main stages.

The first and most primitive stage is characterized by intense aggression and possessiveness of the parents. The aggression is particularly severe in the father and directed mainly to his sons and in the first place to his firstborn son. In early societies it not infrequently culminated in infanticide.

The second stage is caused by a reaction of guilt about aggressive and possessive tendencies and especially about committed infanticide. It results in a compromise solution between the opposing tendencies of the wish to possess the child completely or even to kill him and the desire not to do so. The discovery of the inner laws of this compromise solution was an outstanding achievement of modern psychology. It was the work of Sigmund Freud who called the underlying process the *Oedipus Complex*. The compromise solution of the Oedipus Complex meant moral progress but it created new problems which often tortured the mind more than the previous emotional difficulties.

These mental sufferings can only be overcome when the third stage of moral development of the parent-child relationships is reached. It consists in the entire or almost entire abandonment of possessive, aggressive and especially infanticidal tendencies and their replacement by a covenant of love and affection between parent and child. A process in the direction of this aim was described by Freud as the resolution of the Oedipus complex. It gives admirable insight into important mechanisms at work but cannot explain the essential phenomenon involved and therefore falls short in serving as a guide to achieve the third stage fully. The reason for this lies mainly in the fact that the Oedipus Complex is based on a Greek attitude to life.

New light is thrown on a re-evaluation of the Oedipus Complex and its resolution by a study of parent-child relationships described in the Bible. The Bible contains many stories on this subject but none of them is so important as the story of the sacrifice of Isaac by Abraham. This story is known in Hebrew literature under the name of *The Akedah*.

In the Akedah experience, the third stage of moral development of the parent-child relationships is reached in a completeness as in no other psychological experience.

This study is primarily aimed at a professional audience but is written in a way which can be followed by interested laypersons.

The main object of the study is the description of the Akedah experience and its psychological significance. It is an experience between father and son but its implications affect the whole family and modifications of it occur in all variations of parent-child relationships. In accordance with the three postulated stages of moral development of filio-parental relationships the study is divided into three parts. Part one is an anthropological survey of the aggressive tendencies of primitive parents and especially the custom of infanticide.

The second part describes the psychology of the Oedipus myth and Oedipus Complex. This is done from the viewpoint of the author and has the purpose of preparing the ground for the main theme.

The main theme is rendered in the third part which is devoted to the Akedah. This part expounds theological commentaries, legends and the iconography dealing with the Akedah. The study is based on the observation that phenomena which were described in the Bible occur in every person and provide a unique source for psychological research and insight. It analyses modern psychological theories from the standpoint of Biblical belief. This is the author's approach to psychology. It is his conviction that this approach provides the most satisfactory hypotheses for the motivations in parent-child relationships and thus for human conduct in general.

I

Infanticide

'In Upsal's town the cruel King
Slaughtered his sons at Odin's shrine
Slaughtered his sons with cruel knife
To get from Odin length of life.'

YNGLINGA SAGA

Translated from the Icelandic of Snorro Sturleson by Samuel Laing

Infanticide

THE PRIMAL DEED

'IN the beginning was the deed.' These are the closing words of Sigmund Freud's fundamental book *Totem and Taboo*. In this book he refers to Charles Darwin's hypothesis that in prehistoric times man lived in 'primordial hordes' which were led by a 'primordial father'. Freud assumes that the primordial father was an all-powerful tyrant who owned all women and suppressed and drove away the developing sons. But 'one day the exiled brothers united, killed and ate the father and made an end of his horde'.

Although no evidence exists for Darwin's hypothesis of a primordial horde, Freud's idea of primordial patricide is nevertheless valuable because it suggests that early society passed through a stage of intense conflict between parents and children and especially between fathers and sons.

It is a feature of Freud's psychology that he usually emphasizes the importance of the experiences of the child. This he has also done when he described the hypothetical patricide of the sons. It was, according to his opinion, 'the original sin' of mankind.

Freud did not go into a detailed description of the brutality of the primordial father. But the father's attitude, with that of the mother's, is the first and most formative experience of the children. If one follows up Freud's idea of the primordial father one can, therefore, assume that he not only 'violently and jealously drove away' some of his sons but that he also killed a number of them. This means that before primordial patricide there probably was primordial infanticide. Freud himself noted that the original crime or 'original sin' of mankind is sometimes described in myths as an act of infanticide and not of patricide. The murder and cutting into pieces of the young Dionysos-Zagreus by the first human beings, who were the descendants of the Titans, is an example.

Primitive man expressed his thoughts by deeds. If one considers the possibility of the sons having killed the primordial father one can infer that this was due to the father's behaviour. One can assume that in the beginning was infanticide.

In the beginning of the world, according to Greek cosmogony and theogony, was hatred by the parent of the child and infanticide.

The world of the gods began with Uranus who was created by Gaea, the Earth. Gaea not only was his mother but also his wife. They founded a family of Titans. It was a tragic feature of Greek mythology that Uranus, the primordial father of all Gods, violently hated and cruelly persecuted his children. He did not, however, commit infanticide. This occurred in the second generation.

Cronos, the youngest son of Uranus, with the help of his mother Gaea, rose against the persecution suffered through his father, castrated and dethroned him. His behaviour towards his children was worse than his father's towards him. He initiated infanticide by swallowing his children as soon as they were born and became thus the prototype of the devouring parent. The intensification of the hatred of his children in Cronos as compared with the hatred of Uranus had a particular reason. Cronos was warned by an Oracle that he himself would be supplanted by one of his sons and he knew from his own experience how real this danger was.

In spite of all the precautions of Cronos the Oracle was fulfilled. Zeus, his youngest son, again plotting with his mother, Rhea, overpowered Cronos and became King. The drama of infanticide continued. Zeus was informed that the son which his wife Metis would give him, would banish him from his throne. In order to forestall this he even surpassed his father's actions. He devoured his wife with the embryo in her womb.

These early stories are remarkable, as in their description of filio-parental relationships they foreshadow one of the most mature and moving of all Greek myths: the myth of Oedipus.

THE ANTHROPOLOGY OF INFANTICIDE

Infanticide was practised in historic times all over the world by all races and nations. As will be shown later its character differed greatly according to the societies where it occurred. The following chapter does not claim to be a comprehensive treatment of the subject but will give examples of the relevant material.

Julius Caesar, Suetonius and other ancient writers were appalled by the savagery of human sacrifices and infanticide committed by the French Celts, the Gauls. Children were frequently put to death before battle in order to ensure victory from the gods.[1]

Irish Celts sacrificed children to their God Cromm Cruach,[2] the terrible 'crooked one of the mound'. This was a huge idol which stood on the plain of Magh Sleact, the 'plain of prostrations' in the County of Cavan. It was surrounded by a circle of twelve other idols. The sacrifice took place at

[1] MacCulloch, J. A., 1948. [2] MacCulloch, J. A., 1948.

Samhain, that means at the summer's decline. By pouring their children's blood round the image the parents hoped to obtain an abundance of milk and corn. Firstborn children were sacrificed at the Fair of Taillte in the time of St. Patrick who preached against this.

The Ynglinga Saga, which is the opening part of The Heimskringla, the stories of the Kings of Norway, as told by Snorro Sturleson, an Icelandic chief in the twelfth century, contains many accounts of child murder in ancient Scandinavia.[1] One of them relates how On, King of Sweden, slaughtered nine of his sons in order that Odin might prolong his own life. The moving verses describing this are quoted at the beginning of this chapter.

On's tenth son was Egil. He was rescued from his father's threat by the Swedes and became King. But the wish of his father that he should sacrifice his life for his sake had made a lasting effect on Egil. He only half-heartedly fought against it whilst he was partly willing to obey the father's command. This can be inferred from the story that Egil once hunted a fierce bull and struck him with a spear. The bull probably appeared to Egil as a father figure. The skilful hunter felt unable to complete the kill and so was gored to death by the bull. In this way Egil eventually succumbed to On's father image.

The readiness of the child to be sacrificed at his parent's command plays a great role in the development of filio-parental relationships. It is a tendency which is found in many myths and legends but reached its noblest fulfilment in the attitude of Isaac towards Abraham.

The Spartans in ancient Greece killed their deformed children 'for the good of the state' on the mountain range of Taygetus. The ancient Romans too, forbade by law the rearing of deformed children.

[1] Translated from the Icelandic by Laing, S., 1844.

Infanticide

Infanticide was widely practised amongst the peoples of the Eastern Mediterranean. The Carthaginians slew children 'as if they were lambs or chickens. . . . They placed them one by one, on the sloping hands of the brazen image, from which they rolled into the pit of fire. . . . The mothers had to stand by and see it done without a tear or groan. But all the place in front of the image was filled with a tumultuous music of fifes and drums to drown the shrieks of the victims.'[1] The God to whom the children were sacrificed was variously called Moloch, Melech, Mellsarth or Milcom.

Plutarch[2] stated that Egyptian mothers sacrificed their children to the holy crocodiles and were 'proud' when the children were devoured by the reptiles.

The Pheonicians, according to Porphyry[3], sacrificed their children to Baal.

The Moabites, like all Semetic tribes, followed the custom that in times of great danger their leader should sacrifice his firstborn son as a ransom to the gods. This was described in the Second Book of the Kings.[4] 'And when the King of Moab saw that the battle was too sore for him . . . he took his eldest son that should have reigned in his stead, and offered him for a burnt offering upon the walls.'

The Canaanites who survived the conquest of Palestine by the Israelites used to commit infanticide in order to please their gods. 'Thou shalt not do so unto the Lord thy God' commanded Deuteronomy,[5] 'for every abomination to the Lord, which he hateth, have they done unto their Gods; for even their sons and their daughters they have burnt in the fire to their gods.'

But the Israelites too, at certain periods of their history, relapsed into the customs of the pagans. They made burnt

[1] Plutarch, *De superstitione.* Quoted from Frazer, J. G., 1930.

[2] *Ibid.*

[3] Porphyry, *De abstinentia.*

[4] 2 Kings, iii, 26, 27.

[5] Deuteronomy, xii, 31.

offerings of their children to Baal or Moloch at a place called Tophet. This place was situated in the sinister valley of Hinnom, outside the walls of Jerusalem. The Second Book of Chronicles[1] describes how, in the seventh century B.C., even King Ahaz 'burnt incense in the valley of the son of Hinnom, and burnt his children in the fire, after the abominations of the heathen whom the Lord had cast out before the children of Israel'. In the Second Book of the Kings[2] we read that King Ahaz 'made his son to pass through the fire'. King Manasseh behaved in a similar way.[3]

It is significant that the acts of child sacrifice were equated in the Bible with the worst of all acts of idolatry. In Deuteronomy[4] it is said: 'There shall not be found among you any one that maketh his son or his daughter to pass through the fire, or that useth divination, or an observer of times, or an enchanter, or a witch, or a charmer, or a consultor with familiar spirits, or a wizard, or a necromancer. For all that do these things are an abomination unto the Lord: and because of these abominations the Lord thy God doth drive them before thee'.

Ezekiel[5] linked the slaying of children by the Israelites with the whoredoms and idolatry on high places as child sacrifice was regarded in the Bible with utmost horror.

The prophets therefore fought with all their power against the crime of the Tophet. Three times in the Book of Jeremiah is this fight described. 'And[6] they have built the high places of Tophet . . . to burn their sons and their daughters in the fire. . . . Therefore, behold, the days come, saith the Lord, that it shall no more be called Tophet, nor the valley of the son of Hinnome, but the valley of slaughter; for they shall bury in Tophet, till there be no place. . . .'

[1] 2 Chron., xxviii, 3.
[2] 2 Kings, xvi, 3.
[3] 2 Chron., xxxiii, 6, and 2 Kings, xxi, 6.
[4] Deuteronomy, xviii, 10–12.
[5] Ezekiel, xvi, 20–6.
[6] Jeremiah, vii, 31–4; xix, 5–15; xxxii, 35–6.

Infanticide

'And the carcasses of this people shall be meat for the fowls of the heaven, and for the beasts of the earth; and none shall fray them away.'

'Then I will cause to cease from the cities of Judah, and from the streets of Jerusalem, the voice of mirth, and the voice of gladness, the voice of the bridegroom, and the voice of the bride: for the land shall be desolate.'

Ezekiel said:[1] 'for when ye offer your gifts, when ye make your sons to pass through the fire, ye pollute yourselves. . . .'

Amongst the Arabs the practice of burying children alive, especially little girls, was common. Mohammed forbade this. 'Kill not your children for fear or want.'[2] '. . . the female child that had been buried alive shall be asked [on the Day of Judgement] for what crime she was put to death.'[3]

Infanticide was frequent amongst the negroes of Uganda when the child was the firstborn son of a chief. He was strangled by the midwife immediately after birth and she then reported that 'the child was stillborn'.[4] The West African tribe of the Jagas used to kill all of their children 'because they were a hindrance on the march'.[5] They adopted, however, the adolescent children of parents of other tribes whom the Jagas had killed. This fact makes it likely that the main motive of infanticide was fear of their own children and that the expediency of getting rid of them on a march was largely a rationalization of this fear.

The ancient Mexicans annually sacrificed many children to the Rain God Tlaloc. 'If the children wept it was regarded as a happy omen for a rainy season.'[6]

The Guiana Indians in South America killed especially female and crippled children by breaking their necks, pressing on the breastbone, severing the umbilical cord very near to

[1] Ezekiel, xx, 31.
[2] The Koran. Sura xvii, 33.
[3] The Koran. Sura xxxi, 81.
[4] Frazer, J. G., 1930.
[5] Potter, C. F., 1950.
[6] Spence, L., 1927.

the navel so that the baby must bleed to death, by exposure, or burying the baby alive. The Mbaya women in Brazil killed so many of their children that the nation eventually died out.[1]

Some aborigines in Australia used to kill and eat all firstborn children as part of a religious feast.[2]

Polynesians put a child to death if he resembled the father very much as this was considered as a bad omen for the father.[3] Another reason for infanticide in Polynesia was to reduce the population if food supplies were limited.[4]

The Hindus[5] frequently killed their firstborn children. They were sacrificed to the holy river Ganges by drowning. This custom was in use until the nineteenth century. Another Indian practice was to let the baby suck from his mother's breast which had been anointed with opium.[6]

In his study on *The Religious System of China* J. J. M. De Groat[7] described the occurrence of anthropophagy (cannibalism) and infanticide amongst the Chinese. In the State of Khai-muh, which once existed to the east of Yuch, the firstborn sons used to be killed and devoured. In the realm to the west of Kiao-chi (Tongking) the firstborn sons were chopped into pieces and eaten.

De Groat was at a loss to understand the meaning of this custom which appeared to be so inconsistent with the law of tribal life. He was even 'strongly inclined to believe the statement fabulous'. But from numerous other reports, of which some were given in this study, there can be not the slightest doubt as to the correctness of the statement. As regards the meaning of infanticide, important motives for it existed as will be discussed later.

[1] Potter, C. F., 1950. [2] Smith, R. Brough, 1878.
[3] Potter, C. F., 1950. [4] Frazer, J. G., 1930.
[5] Rose, H. A., Unlucky Children. *Folklore*, xiii (1902). *Indian Antiquary*, xxxi (1902). Quoted from Frazer, J. G., 1930.
[6] Potter, C. F., 1950. [7] De Groat, J. J. M., 1901.

Infanticide

FOUR ASPECTS OF INFANTICIDE

There are four aspects of relationships of parents to their children: the relationships of the mother and father to the son and daughter respectively. In all four aspects, of course, conflicts are bound to arise and infanticide occurred in all of them.

The life-giving principle of motherhood usually was a protective power for the child. But wild passions, ecstasy, frenzy, mad jealousy or sexual and even cannibalistic lust have also driven mothers to kill their children.

The Greek mother Leucippe killed her son Hippasus because she wanted 'to partake of human flesh'.[1]

During the frenzy of Dionysian orgies women used to be seized by such an ecstasy that they tore children apart and devoured the bleeding pieces. These were the sacramental meals called *Omophagy*.[2]

The sinister myth of Medea tells how this unhappy woman in madness through jealousy of her husband Jason slew her three sons. E. S. Stern pointed out[3] that mentally disturbed women not infrequently suffer from infanticidal tendencies and called 'the situation in which the mother harbours death wishes to her offspring' the *Medea Complex*.

Amongst the Chacos Indians of South America the nursing period lasts as long as three to four years during which time women are not allowed to have intercourse. Some of them therefore kill their babies.[4]

In a special category belongs infanticide committed by unmarried mothers because of despair and panic of mind. This is still a not uncommon blemish of our civilization.

[1] Frazer, J. G., 1930.
[2] Farnell, in *The Oxford Classical Dictionary*, 1949.
[3] Stern, E. S., 1948.
[4] Potter, C. F., 1950.

Infanticide

Infanticidal tendencies of the father directed to the daughter, or actually committed infanticide of his daughter by him, are the contents of some of the most moving myths or historical accounts.

In the tale of Troy it is related how the Greek fleet was prevented from sailing because of a dead calm which was brought about by the offended Goddess Artemis. It was announced that Artemis could only be appeased by the sacrifice of King Agamemnon's daughter Iphigenia. The father, after a tragic struggle with himself eventually gave his consent. But when Calchis, the priest, unsheathed his sacrificial knife, Agamemnon could not bear this sight and hid his face. A miracle happened in the last moment and Artemis carried Iphigenia away to her temple in Tauris.

The moving story of Jephtha, the Gileadite, and his daughter ought to be mentioned in this context.[1] Jephtha vowed to the Lord before battle: 'If thou shalt without fail deliver the children of Ammon into mine hands . . . whatsoever cometh forth of the doors of my house to meet me, when I return in peace . . . I will offer it up for a burnt offering.' He conquered the Ammonites and 'his daughter came out to meet him with timbrels and with dances'. And he 'did with her according to his vow which he had vowed'.

This tragedy was caused by the fault of Jephtha. The possibility that his own daughter might be the first one to welcome him ought to have occurred to him before he made the vow. When Jephtha discovered his fault there would have still been a possibility of averting infanticide if he would have recalled and understood the incident of his forefather Abraham's sacrifice of Isaac.

When Othman, the cruel third Caliph, relapsed into the practice of infanticide and buried his little daughter alive 'she reached up her tiny hand and brushed the grave dust

[1] Judges, xi, 30–40.

from his beard'. This was the only instance in Othman's life when he had tears in his eyes.[1]

The relationship between father and son and the conflicts between them are of unique importance. This is due to the fact that human society on the whole has been, and is, a patriarchal one. The patriarchal organization of the family creates special sources of fear and hatred but also of love and affection between the father and his sons and particularly between the father and the firstborn son. Infanticide of the firstborn son committed by the father therefore is an outstanding problem. It is the main subject of this study.

THE MOTIVES OF INFANTICIDE

The fact that infanticide once was a general custom amongst practically all races and nations is a shocking discovery. Many reasons can be given for this sinister fact but all can be reduced to that of selfishness of the parents.

Parenthood involves personal sacrifices for the sake of the child, and indeed, the whole human family. It means renunciation of personal comforts and pleasures. Infanticide committed by mothers was usually due to a craving for gratification of passions. In fathers, the main motive of infanticide was unwillingness to give up their absolute superiority for the benefit of the growing children and particularly the eldest son. These fears were not fleeting emotions, as the passions of the mothers were, but existed continuously. They also struck at the very root of the father's existence and therefore were the most serious cause of infanticide.

The fears of the father were of various kinds. The patriarchal leader feared that he would be overthrown, ousted from his possessions and lose his leadership. This fear was

[1] Frazer, J. G., 1930.

particularly great and real with his natural successor, namely his firstborn son.

Even more tantalizing was the father's fear of being outmatched by his son in his possession of his wife or wives. Incestuous wishes of the son towards his own mother and his desire to possess other wives of his father's clan were a terrible reality.

The greatest danger was the possibility that the son, in order to achieve leadership and possession of women, would kill the father. Patricide, in primitive times, was common although the fathers saw to it that it was less common than infanticide. Patricide, however, was not the only and probably not the most dreaded way in which the father feared to lose his life through his son. A still greater dread was caused by the belief that the father becomes reincarnated in the son.

There was a widespread belief in primitive man that the father is literally reborn in his son. This was especially the case when the son resembled the father in appearance. Some Hindus still believe that the father dies when his son is born and 'in some parts of the Punjab funeral rites are actually performed by the father in the fifth month of his wife's pregnancy'.[1] The belief that the birth of a son means the extinction of the father's life was so revolting and terrifying for many fathers that they killed the son. They could not yet realize that the lives of the father and the son are a unit for the fulfilment of both.

Primitive man must have been conscious to some extent of the true motives of his fears of his son. In order to ease his guilty feelings about his infanticide he rationalized its real motives. He explained the necessity of making a serious sacrifice by plausible reasons but did not admit that it suited his own purpose very well to chose his son as the victim of the sacrifice.

[1] Frazer, J. G., 1930.

The form and moral level of rationalization of infanticide differed greatly amongst the nations. The killing of crippled children 'for the good of the state' or child sacrifice to obtain victory in battle contain altruistic and heroic elements. Rationalizations suggesting that infanticide is necessary in order to limit the numbers in a family or population or necessary to secure a good rainy season and a rich harvest show selfish motives more clearly.

The most important form of rationalization of child murder was the belief that the gods demanded it and were pleased by it. The vicarious sacrifice of the child should cleanse the parents from their sins and show the gods how much they are revered. Infanticide thus was not murder at all but holy sacrifice and a virtuous deed.

According to this rationalization the deed was the more virtuous the greater the danger which the father feared from his child. The danger was greatest with his firstborn son. Therefore infanticide of the firstborn son became the most glorious sacrifice which a father could offer to the gods. This was above all the case when the son was born after many years of childlessness, when he resembled the father closely, and the parents were already advanced in years.

THE MODIFICATIONS OF INFANTICIDE

Infanticide was always a matter of emotional upheaval to the parent. In addition to the rationalization of its true motives another means was found to mitigate the abomination of the deed. It consisted in the modification of its performance.

Originally the killed child probably was eaten. By doing this the parents symbolically incorporated the youthful and envied qualities of the child. It must be reckoned as a sign of moral development when at least cannibalism was given up.

Frazer described this in the natives of Rook, an island near New Guinea. 'They prided themselves in their humanity in burying the murdered infants instead of eating them as their barborous neighbours did.'

The keener the parent was in killing his child the earlier did he do it. Zeus did not take any risks and devoured the embryo even before his birth together with his mother. The fathers in Uganda saw to it that their firstborn sons were killed as soon as they were born. The truth of the gruesome deed, however, was not allowed to be admitted openly and the midwife who strangled the child had therefore to announce that he was stillborn. The longer the child was allowed to live the more opportunities were given to him to escape from his sentence. This must have often been at the back of the parents' mind and especially of that of the mothers. Prolongation of the time when the child sacrifice should be performed meant a dawning hope that the killing might eventually not be carried out.

The most primitive and direct way of killing the child was by the parent's own hand. The child was strangled, suffocated or slain with a knife or another instrument.

A mode to create a symbolically significant distance between the slayer and his victim was to let the child be killed by another power than that of the slayer himself. This was achieved by burning the child in the fire or drowning him in the water. These modes of murdering had also the advantage that no blood had to be shed. In other cases animals were made the direct executioners, as the crocodiles of the river Nile.

A very important modification of the method of committing infanticide, which showed an obvious tendency to avoid it, was the exposure of the infant. The child was usually exposed on the top of a mountain, in a deep forest or in a container which was placed in the sea or river. This widespread custom was a frequent subject of myths and legends.

By not killing the child directly but exposing him to various perils the possibility was left open of an accidental rescue. And, true enough, this secret wish of the parent was not infrequently fulfilled as in the cases of Oedipus and Moses. The theme of the rescue of the exposed child was regarded by ancient tradition as a miraculous happening and the surviving son as a hero who sometimes initiated a new epoch. The effort of the parent to fight his fears, and his secret hope that the child would survive the exposure, marked a new epoch in the moral development of man.

THE QUESTION OF MICAH

Many parents had anxious scruples whether child sacrifice was a virtue after all, able to reconcile and please the offended supernatural power. These scruples were particularly severe amongst the Israelites.

Micah, the Morasthite, the great prophet of the reigns of Jotham, Ahaz and Hezekiah, in his fight against the relapse of Israel into paganism and child murder, asked the challenging question:[1]

Shall I give my firstborn for my transgression,
The fruit of my body for the sin of my soul?

This was a question fundamental not only for Israel but the whole world. There were three answers to the question of Micah.

The first answer was to continue to commit infanticide. The second answer was to stop actual infanticide but to retain infanticidal wishes. The outcome of this was the compromise solution of the Oedipus Complex with its pathological effects.

The third answer had already been given by Micah's ancestor

[1] Micah, vi, 7.

Abraham. Not only must actual infanticide be abolished but also infanticidal wishes. A new relationship must be established between parent and child. This is the meaning of the Akedah. The solution of the Akedah is difficult to achieve but it is the answer to Micah's question on which our mental health and happiness depends.

II

The Oedipus Complex

'King Oedipus, who slew his father Laius and wedded his mother Jocasta, is nothing more or less than a wish-fulfillment, the fulfillment of the wish of our childhood.'

SIGMUND FREUD

The Interpretation of Dreams

The Oedipus Complex

THE COMPROMISE SOLUTION

EVEN during the most primitive and brutal period of history, when man killed some of his children under the pretext that this was his right and even his duty, man's attitude towards infanticide was divided between his desires to kill and to love his child. His brutal selfishness and irrational fear, however, were so overwhelmingly great that infanticide was committed as a matter of course.

The first visible reactions against infanticide were its previously mentioned modifications of disposal of the killed child, timing of the sacrifice, and mode of killing.

The increasing resistance to killing one's own child created the wish that another child should die in his place. This led to the widespread ancient custom that the King's son should be sacrificed as a *vicarious sacrifice* for the community.

Eventually it was realized that any child who was to be sacrificed was actually innocent. But in order to please the gods with some human sacrifice, convicted criminals were vicariously put to death.

Child and other human vicarious sacrifices were eventually abandoned altogether. But the fear and hatred of the young rival and the infanticidal tendencies of the parent still lived on. They now appeared in the parent's desire at least to *injure* or harm his child to give him at least a punishment, a warning, a lesson. This desire was expressed in most interesting customs and ceremonies. Their purpose was to cool down the parent's wrath and thereby to improve his relationship with the child.

The following ceremony was held by Indians of North Carolina down to the eighteenth century.[1]

'The King orders at certain occasions to beat and wound the best beloved of his children with the same weapons wherewith they had been killed in former times, but they are not killed.' The conflict in the King's mind about his order is symbolized by the behaviour of the person who is charged to wound his son. This person 'runs about the house like a distracted person, crying and making the most hideous noise all the time with the weapon in his hand'. The obedience of the King's son is touchingly demonstrated. 'He never offers to stir till he is wounded the third time, after which he falls down backwards stretching out his arms and legs as if he had been ready to expire.' Now the father's aggressive tendencies have abated and he expiates his infanticidal wish. 'Then the King's family and all people fall at their feet and cry and lament most bitterly. The King and his family are feasting but in great silence.' Eventually the victory over the infanticidal wish and the achievement of the compromise is celebrated. 'It follows singing, dancing and great joy.'

Another interesting version of the harming of children who were destined to be sacrificed instead of killing them was reported by Festus and quoted by Frazer.[2] The ancient Italians of Sabine stock, in times of calamity, vowed to sacrifice to the gods all children that should be born in the following spring.

The children, however, were kept alive. When they had

[1] Bricknell, J., *The Natural History of North Carolina*, 1737. Quoted from Frazer, J. G., 1930.

[2] Frazer, J. G., 1930.

grown up sufficiently to be able to fend for themselves they were veiled and driven beyond the boundaries. They were thus made to suffer but their lives were spared.

A further step of moral development as regards the father's aggressive tendencies can be seen in customs which suggest a desire of *the father* to expiate his wish to injure his son by *taking some punishment himself* too. J. Campbell[1] reported the following custom amongst the Crannas of South Africa: 'When the son of a chief has attained manhood his father presents him with a stick. When the son succeeds in knocking his father down he is acknowledged chief of the Kraal.'

In another custom the father, instead of harming the son harmed only himself. He did this by an act of renunciation of his rights. In Tahiti the King, when a son was born to him, abdicated the throne in favour of the infant. The infant's father 'was the first to pay him homage by saluting his feet and declaring him King'. But the father continued to rule as his son's Regent.

In Fiji, 'the father abdicated as soon as the son reached manhood'.

A fascinating phenomenon amongst African natives, which can be interpreted as a self-inflicted deprivation of fathers and an act of expiation for infanticidal wishes, is *La Couvade.* The phenomenon was described by Frazer and analytically studied by Flugel.[2] There is a 'pre-natal' and 'post-natal' Couvade. Before the birth of the child the father will suffer from pains which imitate labour pains. This symbolizes on the one hand love for his wife but on the other hand expiation for his wish to inflict pain on her. After the child's birth the father behaves as if he had been weakened; he lies down in his bed and rejects certain foods. This part of the Couvade

[1] Campbell, J., *Travels in South Africa. Second Journey*. Quoted by Frazer, J. G., 1930.

[2] Flugel, J. G., 1921.

concerns the father's relationship to his child and symbolizes his remorse for his repressed desire to kill the new-born rival. His rejection of food is a sign of his repression of the wish to eat the child.

Although the vicarious injuries of the father represented a moral advance they also supplied a strong incitement to renewed hatred of the child. They were inclined to infuriate the father and stimulate him to take revenge for them. Moral progress was made in the right direction but being not based on a firm conviction of moral values it was not genuine and not enduring.

Another progress in the process of abandoning child sacrifice was its *substitution by an animal sacrifice.*[1] The animals most frequently used were the ram or the lamb. They were a symbolic substitute in the first place for the child but to a certain degree for the father also.

Eventually *no vicarious sacrifice* of any living creature—man or beast—was made *but a mental attitude* assumed which was the outcome of a compromise between infanticidal and love tendencies of the parent. A corresponding attitude of the child also developed, namely a state of compromise between his hate and love impulses towards his parent. The main mental mechanism which produced this psychological state was that of repression of the murderous and hate impulses into the unconscious. In this way the state of mind was developed which Sigmund Freud postulated as the Oedipus Complex. It was named after the Greek myth of Oedipus, King of Thebes.

THE OEDIPUS MYTH

The Oedipus Myth is probably three thousand and possibly four thousand years old.[2] It is likely to be a compilation of

[1] Frazer, J. G., 1930. [2] Pauly, 1916. Robert, 1915.

folklore tales. The main sources of the myth are the Theban Trilogy Oidipodea by Aeschylus, the works Oedipus and Pheonissen by Euripides, and the three Theban plays by Sophocles called 'Oedipus Rex', 'Oedipus at Colonnus' and 'Antigone'.[1]

The Greek genius has developed a particular insight into the tragic conflicts between parents and children. It has produced, besides the Oedipus myth, also the similar and extraordinary legend of Athamas, King of Archaic Orchomenus in Boeotia. Athamas was a variation of Laius and Phrixus, his son, a variation of Oedipus. A ram rescued Phrixus from being sacrificed which is reminiscent of the ram in the story of the sacrifice of Isaac. Frazer described this legend and its bibliography in detail.

Other parallels to the Oedipus myth have been found in various East and North European countries and in other parts of the world.[2]

The main content of the Oedipus myth will now be described. It will be arranged in relation to the three leading figures: Laius, Jocasta and Oedipus.

Laius. When Laius was a young prince he was invited by King Pelops of the Pelopennes to stay with him and teach his son Chrysippos. Laius committed pederasty with Chrysippos and kidnapped him. According to some reports Chrysippos later committed suicide because of his disgrace. Pelops cursed Laius and wished him to remain without child or to die through the hand of his son.

[1] The Sophoclean plays are probably the most widely known source of the myth. Their best-known translation into English was rendered by Jebb (1889; 1893) and were included by P. Mullahy (1948) in his psychological work on the Oedipus myth and complex. The plays have been set in verse by various authors as Gilbert Murray (1948) and E. F. Watling (1946). The verses which will be quoted later are taken from Watling's translation.

[2] *The Standard Dictionary of Folklore, Mythology and Legend*, 1950.

Laius became King of Thebes and married Jocasta, daughter of the Spartan King Menoiceus. According to Sosiphanes[1] Laius killed his father-in-law. This father murder was the second major crime of his life and another omen for his own fate. It was one of the reasons why his marriage with Jocasta was not a happy one.

Laius was much older than Jocasta. When Oedipus met him he described him as an old man with 'silver-frosted hair', whilst Jocasta at that time must have been still relatively youthful.

The marriage remained childless for a long time probably, as Robert[2] assumed, because Laius continued with his pederastic practices. Hera, the Goddess of marriage, was infuriated about this perversion and therefore Appollo's oracle forbade Laius to have a son. Should he beget one, his son would kill him and marry Jocasta. This threat made Laius even more reluctant to have normal intercourse.

A son, however, was born to Jocasta. In spite of the dreaded oracle Laius was reluctant to kill his child. He exposed him on Mount Cithaeron with his feet pierced by a spike and bound together.

The infant was found by a shepherd who brought him to Corinth. King Polybus and Queen Merope of Corinth adopted the child and called him Oedipus, which means 'swollen-footed'.[3] When Oedipus was grown to manhood he was informed by the oracle that he was destined to kill his father and marry his mother. Believing that his adoptive parents were his real parents, Oedipus fled from Corinth.

At the same time Laius set out on a pilgrimage. In a sinister cleft of rocks 'where three roads meet' he encountered a young traveller, who was of the age which his exposed son would have been and who also resembled Laius in his build.

[1] Quoted from Pauly, 1916. [2] Robert, 1915.
[3] Hinsie, L. E., and J. Schatzky, 1940.

Laius was the first to start a quarrel about the right of way. He gave one of his servants a command to thrust Oedipus aside and then struck him on his head with a goad. Did he completely disregard the possibility that the young man might be his surviving son? He certainly did not think of it consciously but there is a strange account from which one can infer that he unconsciously not only considered this but even recognized his son.

In Phoenissen, Euripides reported a version of the fateful meeting on the cross-roads.[1] Oedipus, after he was rudely ordered to go out of the way, at first quietly continued to go on without any act of violence. But then something extraordinary happened: the horses of Laius trod on Oedipus's feet so that they bled. Laius deliberately ordered them to injure Oedipus's feet.[2] He thus ordered for the second time an injury to the feet of 'Swollen-footed'. Oedipus still wore the scars which were caused by the iron spike which pierced his feet. In a flash he too must have unconsciously recognized the father for it was after the injury to his feet that he lost his balance and he tore Laius down from the carriage by his hair and pierced his chest with the sword. Robert[3] gives the illustration on the lid of an antique sacrophagus in the Church of Saint John Lateran in Rome which shows a relief of the scene which was described by Hyginus.

The tragedy of Oedipus was therefore in the last instance actually caused by the defaults of his father Laius. His pederasty, murder of his father-in-law, bad relationship to Jocasta, his cruel order to pierce the baby son's feet, his aggressive behaviour at the cross-roads and his second injury to the son's already scarred feet prepared the catastrophy. But Laius also fought to prevent the impending tragedy. His

[1] Pauly, 1916, and Roscher, W. H., 1897–1902.
[2] Hyginus, C. J., *Fabularum liber*. Quoted from Pauly, 1916.
[3] Robert, 1915.

decision not to kill the son but to expose him proved that he unconsciously wished that he might survive. His last journey was a 'pilgrimage'. It is not stated what its purpose was but it is not unjustified to conjecture that Laius, in constant thought of his only son, wanted to expiate his guilt.

Jocasta. After his patricide Oedipus came to Thebes. The city was at that time overcome by a great calamity. Hera, in order to punish the Thebans because they condoned the pederasty of their king sent them a monster, the Sphinx, which destroyed all who could not answer her riddle. Oedipus solved her riddle and as a reward received the Kingdom of Thebes and the widowed Queen Jocasta as his wife.

Jocasta, after her unhappy marriage with the old and perverted Laius, probably was looking forward to wed the young hero. This desire must have dimmed her judgement of the situation. For Oedipus was just of the same age which her son would have been if he had still been alive. He also resembled Laius in his figure. No definite proof of the actual death of her exposed baby son ever reached her and, what mother, in these circumstances, would have ever given up hope that her son had survived and that she might perhaps one day see him again? The oracle said that she would and prophecies of the oracle in ancient Greece were generally believed to come true.

But there was a still more serious sign which ought to have made her suspicious of her husband-to-be. This was his name Oedipus, 'Swollen-footed'. True enough, Oedipus himself did not know the exact origin of his name. But Jocasta knew that her baby son had been exposed and she most likely knew that his feet had been pierced. Even if she should not have known that his feet had been pierced she was acquainted with the custom of her time of driving a spike through the feet of a person whom one wishes to prevent from escaping to safety.

There was a simple way for Jocasta to investigate the possible origin of the name of Oedipus: to inspect his ankles. They still showed the old scars.[1] They must have made it likely to Jocasta that Oedipus was exposed as a baby. But Jocasta did not investigate. This was her guilt.

She married Oedipus and had by him two sons and two daughters. But the gods to whom nothing was hidden punished the city because of what occurred within its walls. The plague broke out and Thebes was on the verge of extinction. The oracle declared that the peril could only be averted by tracing and punishing the murderer of Thebes' former king, Laius.

This is the moment when the play 'Oedipus Rex' by Sophocles begins. Driven by a mysterious urge Oedipus solemnly cursed the unknown murderer and embarked on a relentless search for him. Step by step he came nearer to the truth.

Jocasta was seized by a sinister foreboding. She was well acquainted with the existence of incestuous tendencies in men directed to the mother and strenuously tried to dispel Oedipus's growing suspicion. She said to him that he need not be frightened by his fear that he might have married his mother because:

> *Many a man has dreamt as much*
> *Such things must be forgotten,*
> *If life is to be endured.*

The more she herself became afraid of the outcome of the inquiry the more she fought heroically to save her husband and her child. When Tiresias, the seer, eventually pronounced the truth, Jocasta hanged herself, expiating her tragic life as a Greek heroine.

Oedipus. Like many adopted children who have not been told of the fact of their adoption, Oedipus still probably had a

[1] Hyginus, C. J. *Ibid.*

feeling of uncertainty about his origin. When, at a feast, a drunken man actually told him that Polybus and Merope were not his real parents, he was tortured by this statement. He implored Polybus and Merope to tell him the truth but they denied the drunken man's story so unconvincingly that Oedipus secretly asked the oracle. The oracle, however, did not answer his question at all. But it sent him to his horror the message that he was destined to kill his father and marry his mother. He was panic-stricken. Polybus and Merope could have been his true parents after all. He fled from Corinth.

But on the other hand the oracle did not reassure him as to his true origin and he must have reckoned with the possibility that his real parents might be unknown to him. Why then, was Oedipus not careful in his approach to the old man whom he met on the cross-roads, and who, according to age could have been his father? Why did he not flee from the scene of the quarrel as he fled from Corinth? As a matter of fact, the thought of asking the old man if he were his father actually occurred to him unconsciously, in a fleeting moment. This is revealed in 'Oedipus at Colonnus' when he said to Creon:

> *If here and now*
> *Someone came up and threatened to take your life,*
> *Your innocent life,*
> *Would you then pause to ask if he were your father—*
> *Or deal with him out of hand?*

Oedipus did not pause to ask. He unconsciously did not care to ask but cared to kill.

Nor did Oedipus recoil from marrying Jocasta, although he could not have been sure that Merope was his real mother. If he believed the inescapable prediction of the oracle then he would on no account have married any woman who was so much older than himself that she could have been his mother.

Maddened by horror about the final disclosures Oedipus blinded himself with the golden brooches of Jocasta's garment.

After these events the suffering of Oedipus continued in his relationship to his children. It is remarkable that he did not show much concern about his sons Polynices and Eteocles, and that in his behaviour towards them he repeated the aggressive attitude of Laius against himself. When he made his last will after his blinding he said to Creon:

> *Don't trouble yourself about the boys, Creon:*
> *They will be able to fend for themselves*
> *Wherever they go.*

That they were not able to fend for themselves their tragic future showed. It seems as if they were always lacking in their father's love. This explains much of their revolt against him. In order to show him their disrespect they sent him a bad piece of sacrificial meat; they imprisoned him, giving as pretext for this deed the need to hide him from the world because of his disgrace.[1] When a rebellion broke out in Thebes and King Oedipus was expelled his sons refused to help him. Oedipus' reaction towards their unfaithfulness was terrible. He cursed them and the curse came true.

Oedipus's daughters Antigone and Ismene on the other hand were his 'darlings'. They took his side when he was expelled from Thebes. The story seems to imply that there was an incestuous element in his love towards them, especially to Antigone. Although there was, perhaps, some justification in the wish that his daughters should not marry because of the scandal of their birth, this wish might have coincided with his selfish desire to tie them nearer to him.

[1] Robert, C., 1915.

Antigone in particular reciprocated the excessive emotional bond. She led the blind father on his way to exile. She resembled him strikingly in heroism, readiness for sacrifice, and liability to raging temper outbursts. After her father's death she vehemently wished to see his grave although this was taboo. As the play 'Antigone' shows, her love for her brother Polynices had an incestuous flavour. Oedipus's problems lived on in his children.

Oedipus was a hero of suffering. His relentless search for truth and desire for expiation gave him sacredness. His sacrifices were so moving because they were felt to be vicarious for the potential crimes of others. The piercing of his feet is strangely reminiscent of the wounding of the Suffering Servant in Isaiah liii and the piercing of Jesus' feet on Golgotha. In his repentance and expiation he wished to return to Mount Cithaeron in order to die there 'obedient to his parents' original desire'.

As a sign in his outstanding virtues Oedipus was distinguished by dying a death unlike that of any ordinary mortal. On his wanderings he eventually reached Colonnus near Athens. There he mysteriously disappeared on a hilltop in the sacred grove of the Eumenides like a semi-god.

Oedipus had struggled in a heroic and saintly manner. But the outcome of his struggle was a compromise with a tragic end and did not reach a redeeming solution.

THE OEDIPUS COMPLEX

Sigmund Freud's discovery of the Oedipus Complex is related to experiences which he gained during his own childhood.[1] He was the firstborn son of a youthful mother who had a religious trust in his future destiny. His father was twenty years older than his mother. Sigmund revered him 'as the wisest man' but also hated him. His father was critical

[1] Helen Walker-Puner, 1949.

and once said that 'that boy (Sigmund) will not amount to anything'. Sigmund was also deeply disappointed because his father did not represent to him the ideal of Jewish-Semitic greatness. This ideal he had formed in himself under the influence of his mother, the descendant of a great Talmudic scholar and from the study of the history of Hannibal, the great Semitic conqueror. So painful was the disappointment of his love for his father that it is not impossible that his father's death meant the relief of a tension in him which released his greatest creative powers. For it was soon after his father's death, in 1900, that he published his perhaps greatest work: *Die Traumdeutung*, *The Interpretation of Dreams*.

In this visionary work the Oedipus Complex was described for the first time. Freud began the description of this phenomenon by emphasizing the strange fact that a modern reader or playgoer is not less powerfully moved by the extraordinary content of the Oedipus Rex than were the contemporaries of Sophocles. And then he enunciated these sentences which shook the world:

'There must be a voice within us which is prepared to acknowledge the compelling power of fate in the Oedipus. And there actually is a motive in the story of King Oedipus which explains the verdict of this inner voice. His fate moves us only because it might have been our own. . . . It may be that we were all destined to direct our first sexual impulses toward our mothers and our first impulses of hatred and resistance toward our fathers.'[1]

The fundamental fact that parents and children not only love each other but inevitably also unconsciously harbour hatred and incestuous desires between each other Sigmund Freud postulated as the Oedipus Complex. It became a corner-stone not only for the understanding of filio-parental relationships but also of modern psychology as a whole.

[1] Freud, S., *The Interpretation of Dreams*.

The Oedipus Complex

The Development of the Oedipus Complex. The Oedipus Complex is a phenomenon which is closely linked with the mental and biological development of the child. The first period of a child's life is a state of paradisiacal harmony between him and his parents. Freud[1] described the emotional filio-parental relationship prior to the development of the Oedipus Complex. The infant boy, during this period, wishes to be like his father. The father is his ideal. He identifies himself with him. The motives of this phenomenon are the son's admiration of his father, his need for protection and desire to take possession of him which he achieves by the mechanism of *Identification.* At the same period the son also develops a primal tender love for his mother. This is due to his realization of his dependence on her care and love, and on her breast, as the organ which is symbolic for these greatest of all feelings.

The beginning and further development of the Oedipus Complex can be best studied in the light of *the psycho-sexual development of the child* as taught by Freud. Psycho-analytic theory provides a coherent account of the mental development of the child. It distinguishes bio-psychological phases which are of essential importance for the understanding of normal and pathological psychology of the child and the adult.

Already during the first year of his life the first clouds of conflicts between the child and the parents arise. During this year the most important excitations of the child are centred around the mouth and consist in sucking and biting. It is the *oral phase.* In the boy his tender love towards his mother gradually assumes the character of possessive sensuous wishes. He also learns that his father is a hindrance to these wishes and commences to hate him although, at the same time, he continues to love him. This is the setting in which the Oedipus Complex grows and develops.

[1] Freud, S., *Group Psychology and Analysis of the Ego*, 1922.

The Oedipus Complex

It is significant that the opposing love and hate tendencies of the son towards his father, which mark the beginning of the Oedipus situation, have a parallel in the development of opposing emotions during the oral phase: the intake of food on the one hand means an act of loving union with the mother but on the other hand aggression towards the food. The sucking on the breast is a pleasurable experience but if the child is hungry he will punish the breast by biting it.

During the second year *anal-urethral* excitations dominate. They also are of an oppositional character, consisting in the tendencies to retain or to expel products of metabolism.

As from the third year, *genital* excitations steadily increase. They reach their climax in the fifth and sixth year. The child becomes aware of his genitals. He becomes interested in the differences between boys and girls, the mystery of birth, and, above all, in the intimacy between his parents.

It is during this genital phase of psycho-sexual development that the Oedipus Complex mainly develops. In the son, sensuous love towards his mother and hatred towards his father are at its height. Parallel with these impulses he develops a fear of retaliation by being castrated, which has been termed the *Castration Complex.*[1] These emotions, however, exist together with tender feelings for both parents. Therefore the child is in one of the most difficult and dangerous periods of his life.

The Elements of the Oedipus Complex. The Oedipus Complex is characterized by the existence of incestuous and hate impulses on one side and of tender love impulses on the other. These elementary factors build up the intricate and complicated phenomenon of the complex.

The most shocking aspect of the Oedipus Complex is the repulsive disclosure of the existence of *incestuous tendencies* between children and parents. It was on this issue that Freud's

[1] Abraham, K., 1949.

doctrine was mainly attacked or modified. Some of the critics furnished very valuable additional insight into the Oedipus phenomenon.

A. Adler,[1] conforming with the popular rejection of the incest motive, explained the Oedipus situation as an urge for power which occurs, for instance, in sons who were excessively pampered, kissed and caressed by their mothers. C. Jung[2] explained the incest wish as a symbol which may mean the desire to withdraw from the difficult reality of this world and to return to the womb and bliss of the infant. The longing for the body of the mother may also mean a striving towards communion with infinite life. O. Rank[3] thought that the incest urge is the melancholy wish to escape from the hardship of life and return into the womb of the mother, which is the 'paradise lost' of man. S. Ferenczi,[4] like Jung, also believed in a symbolic aspect of the Oedipus theme. But, unlike Jung, he laid greater stress on the actual sexual significance of the Oedipus situation. He also pointed out that the heroic desire of Oedipus to find out the truth is symbolic of an equally heroic desire in ourselves to bring dark, unconscious facts into the light of consciousness. Also H. Silberer believed in the co-existence of a sexual and symbolic element in the Oedipus phenomenon. The symbolic element is an expression of man's moral and religious strivings. He termed it the *anagogic* element of the Oedipus Complex.

Another shocking aspect of the Oedipus Complex is the finding that, contrary to popular belief, parents and children inevitably harbour *hate impulses* against each other. Hatred and aggression are an innate primary urge which, as Anna Freud[5] has said, existed since the beginning of life. In primitive times the hate impulses of parents towards their children

[1] Adler, A., 1938.
[2] Jung, C., 1919.
[3] Rank, O., 1926.
[4] Ferenczi, S., 1926.
[5] Freud, Anna, 1947.

led to the custom of infanticide and not infrequently also to patricide. There are authors like E. Fromm[1] and O. Rank[2] who consider the aggressive tendencies between father and son to be the predominant factor in the Oedipus situation.

On the other side of the incestuous and hate impulses of the Oedipus Complex operate the *tender love impulses* between children and parents. They are an innate primary force of the psyche and have brought about the phenomenon of identification of the child with his parent at the beginning of life. This phenomenon becomes reinforced and modified during the development of the Oedipus situation as a curative reaction against the increasing difficulties of the Oedipus conflict.

The essence of the Oedipus Complex consists in the *simultaneous operation of hate and incestuous impulses* on the one *and tender love impulses* on the other side. The co-existence of two contradictory feelings of wishes was termed by the Swiss psychiatrist, Bleuler, *ambivalence*. The son, for instance, wants to express his hatred for the father but, as the same time, he also feels a tender love for him.

As man's moral development progresses, the hate impulses are more and more repressed into the unconscious whilst the tender love impulses remain in the light of consciousness. This is the reason why Freud's discovery of the Oedipus Complex came as a distasteful challenge to popular opinion.

The repressed hate impulses live on in the unconscious mind and continuously urge for satisfaction. The conflicting hate and love tendencies create a torturing tension which demands relief. It is brought about by a compromise between the conflicting forces.

The Variations of the Oedipus Theme. In the case of the son, he tends to develop an ambivalent relationship to his father and to his mother only a tender, libidinous relationship. This

[1] Fromm, E., 1948, 1952. [2] Rank, O., 1926.

condition is the *Simple or Positive Oedipus Complex*. The corresponding mechanism applies to the daughter. In its pure form it occurs only rarely.

Far more common is a more complicated state of affairs. It is caused by the bi-sexual nature of man, that is by the fact that every person, child or adult, possesses to some degree features of both sexes. The boy, therefore, may behave in certain ways like a girl. He may in this case develop to some extent a tender relationship to his father and a jealous and hostile one to his mother. This condition is the *Complete or Negative Oedipus Complex*. It is found in varying degrees in the majority of persons and characteristically occurs in most neurotics.

The Oedipus Complex is a combination of love and hate impulses which are unconsciously acting between all members of the family. There therefore exist a number of *Sub-Complexes of the Oedipus Complex*. These sub-complexes can also be named from Greek mythology. One can distinguish a *Laius*, *Jocasta* and *Oedipus Sub-Complex*. As this study emphasizes, the Laius Sub-Complex is a basic aspect of the whole Oedipus situation. The sub-complex of the daughter was termed by Jung[1] the *Electra Complex*.

Other sub-complexes of the manifold variations of the Oedipus theme can also be distinguished. When the hatred of the son's feminine aspect is directed against his mother the condition can be termed the *Orestes Complex*.[2] The mother's hatred of her son, which originates from her male aspect, was termed by E. S. Stern[3] the *Medea Complex*.

[1] Jung, C. G., 1917. Electra was the daughter of the Greek king Agamemnon who was murdered by his wife Clytemnestra. Electra's devotion to her father was as great as her hatred of her mother.

[2] Orestes, with the help of his sister Electra, murdered his mother Clytemnestra as revenge for her murder of his father Agamemnon.

[3] Stern, E. S., 1948. Medea killed her children in an attack of mad jealousy.

The Oedipus Complex

Freud used the term Oedipus Complex for all combinations of its variations showing the emphasis he placed on the sub-complex of the child and in particular the son. The reasons for this lie in Freud's own childhood experiences and in the developmental approach of his teaching.

The Oedipus Complex is of prime importance not only for the understanding of normal but also of pathological psychology. According to a dictum of Freud[1] it not only is one amongst other complexes causing a neurosis but even is 'the nuclear complex of the neurosis'. This means that the Oedipus Complex, as it were, stands in the centre of all neurotic disturbances.

This can be most clearly seen in conversion hysteria. This psycho-neurosis is caused by a frustration of incestuous impulses mainly experienced during the genital phase of the psycho-sexual development of the child, that is during the phase when the Oedipus conflict is at its height.

The Heir of the Oedipus Complex. Normally the five- or six-year-old child realizes that his hate and incestuous impulses were wrongly-displayed emotions and incompatible with his happiness. This mental discovery goes parallel with a steady decrease of genital impulses. It is the sign that the Oedipus Complex and with it the castration fear is gradually resolved. The process of *the resolution of the Oedipus Complex* is of greatest importance. On it the mental health of a person depends.

The resolution of the Oedipus Complex changes the personality fundamentally. It is brought about by the emergence of a new psychological force: the *Super-Ego*.[2]

The super-ego is a force which desensualizes libidinous and inhibits aggressive impulses. It controls these impulses and therefore is a moral force. When fully developed it will dominate the psyche as the Oedipus Complex has done be-

[1] Freud, S., 1949.

[2] Freud, S., 1927, The Ego and the Super-Ego in *The Ego and the Id.*

fore. It is in the words of Freud: 'the heir of the Oedipus Complex.'

Although it is not fully developed before the fifth or sixth year the first origins of the super-ego can be traced back to the oral and anal phrases of the child's life. Its full development takes place normally during the genital phase, that is, during the period when the Oedipus Complex grows to its greatest intensity.[1]

The first event in the process of the emergence of the super-ego is the child's desire to change his present unhappy attitude towards his parents. He is desirous to return to the happy state of filio-parental relationship which existed at the beginning of his life. He therefore *reinforces his old identifications* with the parents which became weakened by the storms of the Oedipus conflict.

The regained wish of the child to be like the parents leads him to the desire to incorporate the mental pictures which he formed of them into his own psyche. This process is called *Introjection.* By introjecting the mental pictures of his parents the child uses his parents less and less as targets for his aggressive and incestuous impulses. The introjected parental images include the moral attitudes of the parents. They now become part of the child's own ego. His ego will thus be transformed. The transformed new part of the ego is the super-ego.

The introjected images of the parents contain the parents' own super-egos which, in turn, have been formed by the super-egos of their forefathers. In this way the super-egos of the human race are introjected into a child. This view comes near to Jung's postulation of a racial or collective unconscious and of archetypes.

The introjected moral standards of the parents form an ideal in the child's ego or an *ego-ideal* towards which he

[1] Glover, E., 1949.

strives. This ideal has become part of himself and he loves it with a love which is directed no longer towards his parents but towards himself.

Self-love is called *narcissism*. There existed a primitive narcissism in the child before the development of the super-ego. It was directed towards his self as it originally was and is called *primary narcissism*. The narcissism which develops during the super-ego formation is directed towards the newly erected ego-ideal of the introjected parent images. It is a sublime form of self-love and is termed *secondary narcissism*. The libido which formerly was directed towards the parents becomes desensualized. It now flows towards the self and in this way becomes sublimated.

As a moralizing force the super-ego has powerful effects. It represents the moral code of the parents, forefathers and society. It admonishes, commands, demands expiation and punishment and can be of great severity and even of destructive cruelty.

The super-ego, by imposing its laws on the ego, often finds itself in a state of severe conflict with the ego. In order to lower the painful tension between the super-ego and ego a compromise is made between them. The super-ego, instead of completely suppressing the aggressive and incestuous urges, allows the ego to indulge in them for a while and in a mitigated form. For this concession, however, the ego has to pay dearly. For the super-ego soon replaces the temporary allowance given by the original severe prohibitions which created a state of torture in the ego. The process of re-enacting and the forbidding of the primitive desires is repeated over and over again.[1] The super-ego in this process is a sadistic and the ego a masochistic force. The term given to the process is *moral masochism*. It represents a perpetual repeti-

[1] Glover, E., 1949.

tion of the compromise solution of the Oedipus Complex and often lends to mental breakdown.

The super-ego, through *instinct transformation*, relegates intolerable ideas of hatred and incest from consciousness into the unconscious so that they are now 'forgotten' and become inactive. This fundamental mental mechanism is called *repression*. Some 'forbidden' ideas are consciously turned into opposite, morally approved values, by the process of *reaction formation*. Intolerable thoughts may also be 'cast out' or *projected* into the environment. Other primitive desires may be *displaced* from forbidden aims to permissible ones. The approved aims may be of scientific, artistic or religious value. In this case the displacement is a *sublimation*.

THE CURSE OF THE COMPROMISE SOLUTION

The essence of the Oedipus Complex is the ambivalent value of its elements and the compromise solution of their conflicts. In this compromise each of the opposing forces gives up part of its demands. The tender love impulses, as it were, agree that some hate impulses may be realized. The hate impulses agree to modify their aims.

A compromise solution, however, is fraught with dangers. It only temporizes the actual issue without clearly solving it. It keeps man in a state of perpetual unrest and prevents him from fulfilling his full moral task.

The danger of this torturing and crippling state lies in the fact that there exists a strong tendency for the compromise actions of the Oedipus Complex to give way more and more to the primitive forces of hatred and incestuous desire. This tendency is the main cause of psychological suffering and disease.

The filio-parental relationships which are usually encountered are the result of the compromise solution of the Oedipus

Complex. The relationships are superficially balanced and practically workable but under stress they easily break down. In order to prevent mental breakdown a clear and redeeming solution of the Oedipus Complex is needed.

The despair about the absence of such a solution was movingly expressed by the poet A. E. Housman in 'A Shropshire Lad'.[1] In this work he describes a wish to be dead so that there would be no longer torture by the sin of the father and by the mother's curse. Although Housman's verses were written in a depressed mood, their content is nevertheless characteristic for what countless people vaguely feel. The verses terminate with the sinister vision of a curse. With the intuition of the poet, Housman expressed the very judgement of the hero of the Oedipus myth about the cause of his suffering.

The deepest reason for the tragedy of Oedipus lay not in his misfortune of committing crimes which he did not will, and even strenuously fought, but in his inability to find a redeeming solution of his inner conflicts. All he was able to achieve was a compromise between his conflicting impulses. There was something missing in all his valiant and even saintly efforts. There was a tragic lack of insight and moral decision in his thoughts and actions. This was due to his lack of a guiding vision, which was symptomatic of the Greek tragic view of life. Oedipus himself felt that the solution which he found was insufficient and the cause of his suffering. He did not have the insight to express this clearly but in his tortured mind he had the intuition to call his failure a curse. Immediately following his discovery that he himself killed his father he spoke these words:

On me is the curse that none but I have laid.

The tragedy of Oedipus was perpetuated in his relation-

[1] Housman, A. E., 1916.

ship to his sons Polynices and Eteocles. When they betrayed him he cursed them with a terrible curse. He said to Polynices, his firstborn son, these words in which one already can hear approaching madness:

> *. . . you shall fall,*
> *You and your brother, with blood on both your hands,*
> *I cursed you once before; I curse you now.*

'The curse of his sons', said Gilbert Murray,[1] 'made Oedipus a hero of suffering in the eyes of the Greeks, for how otherwise could he have acted and how did he himself suffer by doing it?' It was indeed the tragedy of Oedipus that he did not know what otherwise he could have done. The feeling deep in his conscience that there existed a solution which, however, he could not find, drove him to madness.

The unbearable state of an unsatisfactory compromise solution of the Oedipus situation maddened also other mythological or legendary heroes, as for instance King Athamas and King Lear. In primitive customs too, which were connected with the actual or symbolic sacrifice of a son, madness was acted. Frazer[2] mentioned examples of these customs amongst the natives of Peru and North Carolina. This significantly shows that in the minds of ancient and primitive people, as in the vision of the poet, madness is a not infrequent outcome of the unsatisfactory solution of the Oedipus Complex.

Sigmund Freud spoke of the Oedipus conflict as of a curse which was laid upon man. In his postulation of the Oedipus Complex he said:[3]

'His (Oedipus's) fate moves us only because it might have been our own, because the oracle laid upon us before our birth the very curse which rested upon him.'

But the curse is not simply inherited. It is also acquired by

[1] Murray, G., 1948. [2] Frazer, J. G., 1930. [3] Freud, S., 1900.

the actions of each person. For these each individual bears responsibility.

The deepest reason for the curse is not given by the poem, myth or psychological dictum quoted but by the Bible. So important is its issue that it was given at an extraordinary place in the Bible, namely in the last verses of the last of the prophets. There Malachi said:[1]

'Behold, I will send you Elijah the prophet before the coming of the great and dreadful day of the Lord:

'And he shall turn the heart of the fathers to the children, and the heart of the children to their fathers, lest I come and smite the earth with a curse.'

The immense importance of these verses is shown by the fact that they reappear in a variation at the beginning of the New Testament.[2] In Luke,[3] the angel said to Zecharia when he annunciated the birth of John the Baptist:

'And he shall go before him in the spirit and power of Elias, to turn the hearts of the fathers to the children, and the disobedient to the wisdom of the just; to make ready a people prepared for the Lord.'

Malachi and Luke pointed to the central significance of the victory of the tender lover over the aggressive and incestuous tendencies in parents and children. But they said more than that. They emphasized that the 'turning of the heart' is a command which was given to us by a divine power outside ourselves and that on the obedience or disobedience to it all human future and happiness depends. But, so far, the hearts of most fathers and children have not yet turned to each other. And therefore the Lord has smitten the earth with a curse: the curse of selfishness, violence and greed.

The unsatisfactory compromise solution of the Oedipus Complex is not an inevitable issue. It can be turned into a clear and full solution, as a curse can be turned into a bless-

[1] Malachi, iv, 5, 6. [2] Quandt, E., 1871. [3] Luke, i, 17.

ing, if the appropriate attitude of mind is adopted. This attitude has been described in the Bible in the phenomenon of the *Akedah.* The significance of the solution of the Akedah for modern man lies in the fact that it can be repeated in everybody.

III

The Akedah

'And he said,
Lay not thine hand upon the lad,
neither do thou any thing unto him.'

GENESIS, XXII, 12

'And in thy seed shall all the nations
of the earth be blessed;
because thou hast obeyed my voice.'

GENESIS, XXII, 18

The Akedah

THE MEANING OF THE AKEDAH

THE *Akedah* or *Akeedath Yitzhac* means 'The Binding of Isaac'.[1] The expression is derived from the First Book of Moses or Genesis, chapter xxii, verse 9:

'And Abraham built an altar . . . and bound Isaac his son.'

The Hebrew word *Akad* means 'to bind', in particular the bent fore and hind legs of an animal which is destined for sacrifice. The word occurs in the Old Testament only in the verse quoted above.[2] The expression of *the Akedah* signifies the event of Abraham's attempted but averted sacrifice of Isaac as it was related in the first nineteen verses of the twenty-second chapter of Genesis. Almost every word in this extraordinary story is of importance for this study and therefore the story is quoted below in full.[3]

'And it came to pass after these things, that God did tempt Abraham, and said unto him, Abraham: and he said, Behold, here I am.

2 And he said, Take now thy son, thine only son Isaac, whom thou lovest, and get thee into the land of Moriah; and offer him there for a burnt offering upon one of the mountains which I will tell thee of.

[1] Hershon, P. I., 1885.
[2] Driver, S. R., 1906.
[3] The Authorized Version of the Holy Bible is used.

The Akedah

3 And Abraham rose up early in the morning, and saddled
his ass, and took two of his young men with him, and
Isaac his son, and clave the wood for the burnt offering,
and rose up, and went unto the place of which God had
told him.
4 Then on the third day Abraham lifted up his eyes, and
saw the place afar off.
5 And Abraham said unto his young men, Abide ye here
with the ass; and I and the lad will go yonder and worship,
and come again to you.
6 And Abraham took the wood of the burnt offering, and
laid it upon Isaac his son; and he took the fire in his hand,
and a knife; and they went both of them together.
7 And Isaac spake unto Abraham his father, and said, My
father: and he said, Here am I, my son. And he said, Be-
hold the fire and the wood: but where is the lamb for a
burnt offering?
8 And Abraham said, My son, God will provide himself a
lamb for a burnt offering: so they went both of them
together.
9 And they came to the place which God had told him of;
and Abraham built an altar there, and laid the wood in
order, and bound Isaac his son, and laid him on the altar
upon the wood.
10 And Abraham stretched forth his hand, and took the
knife to slay his son.
11 And the angel of the Lord called unto him out of heaven,
and said, Abraham, Abraham: and he said, Here am I.
12 And he said, Lay not thine hand upon the lad, neither
do thou any thing unto him: for now I know that thou
fearest God, seeing thou hast not withheld thy son, thine
only son from me.
13 And Abraham lifted up his eyes, and looked, and behold
behind him a ram caught in a thicket by his horns: and

Abraham went and took the ram, and offered him up for a burnt offering in the stead of his son.
14 And Abraham called the name of that place Jehovah-jireh: as it is said to this day, In the mount of the Lord it shall be seen.
15 And the angel of the Lord called unto Abraham out of heaven the second time,
16 And said, By myself have I sworn, saith the Lord, for because thou hast done this thing, and hast not withheld thy son, thine only son:
17 That in blessing I will bless thee, and in multiplying I will multiply thy seed as the stars of the heaven, and as the sand which is upon the sea shore; and thy seed shall possess the gate of his enemies;
18 And in thy seed shall all the nations of the earth be blessed; because thou hast obeyed my voice.
19 So Abraham returned unto his young men, and they rose up and went together to Beer-sheba; and Abraham dwelt at Beer-sheba.'

THE THEOLOGICAL IMPORTANCE OF THE AKEDAH

The story of the Akedah is one of many deeply meaningful stories in the Bible but seems to describe the fundamental event on which the whole Bible stands. Its inner meaning is basic to religious development of Judaism and Christianity and also plays a dominant role in Islam.

The Akedah in Judaism. The Akedah is an important subject of Jewish folklore and legends, many of which are based on ancient tradition. This tradition is known as *Haggada* and is contained in the *Talmud* and the *Midrashim.*[1] It added many

[1] *Midrasch Rabba.* Translated into English under the editorship of H. Freeman, 1939; *Der Midrasch Bereschit Rabba.* Translated into German by A. Wuensche.

stories and commentaries to the Bible, some of them being of a fantastic, others of a speculative nature, but most of them being derived from the depths of Jewish religiosity.[1]

During the Middle Ages the Akedah obtained a prominent place in Jewish Liturgy. This was caused by the horrors of persecution of the Jewish faith of this time. The Akedah was held up as an example of devotion in faith and its merit was invoked when appeals were made for God's mercy. During this time numerous Akedah prayers were composed in stirring, poetical language.[2]

In some rites the Akedah chapter is read daily as part of the morning service.[3] On the Jewish New Year's Day the complete story of the Akedah is read out of the Scroll of the Torah with the greatest solemnity. The Akedah is commemorated in the Musaf-Tefilla of this day.[4]

The New Year's Day is the Day of Judgement and as such the precursor of the Day of Atonement which is celebrated ten days after the New Year. Judgement and atonement are both related to the Akedah.[5] This is expressed by the blowing of the *shofar*, that is the horn of a ram, on New Year's Day.[6] When Rabbi Abbahu was asked why the shofar should be sounded he answered: 'Because God said: Sound before Me the ram's horn so that I may remember on your behalf the binding of Isaac, the son of Abraham, and account it to you as if you had bound yourselves before Me.'[7]

The Akedah in Christianity. As Christianity has at its centre

[1] Ginzberg, L., 1909; Micha Josef bin Gorion, 1914.

[2] Dukes, L., 1842; Zunz, 1855, mentioned about thirty authors of such prayers or poems, most of which were written in Hebrew.

[3] Gaster, N., 1928; *The Festival Prayers according to the Ritual of the German and Polish Jews*, 1876; Asher, D., 1866.

[4] Zunz, 1855.

[5] Pesitka, quoted from Zunz, 1855.

[6] Maimonides, Yad Shofar, Shulhan Aruk, Orah Hayyim. Quoted from *The Jewish Encyclopedia*, 1925.

[7] Babylonian Talmud. Rosh Hashana, 16a.

the Sacrifice of Jesus, the Sacrifice of Isaac must also occupy a central place.

In the *Epistle of James*,[1] James, the brother of Jesus and first Bishop of Jerusalem said: 'Was not Abraham our father justified by works, when he had offered Isaac his son upon the altar?' James in the passage emphasized that Abraham not only meditated about what he ought to do but actually carried out the command of God.

The writer of the *Epistle to the Hebrews*[2] said: 'By faith Abraham, when he was tried, offered up Isaac: and he that had received the promises offered up his only begotten son, Of whom it was said, That in Isaac shall thy seed be called: Accounting that God was able to raise him up, even from the dead; from whence also he received him in a figure.'

The analogy of the Akedah with the Sacrifice of Jesus is so striking that the Church Fathers[3] frequently referred to it.

For the same reason the Sacrifice of Isaac plays an important role in Christian Liturgy.

In the Church of England on Good Friday the First Lesson is the Akedah (Genesis, xxii, 1–19). The Second Lesson on that day is fittingly St. John, xviii, the chapter of the beginning of the drama of Golgotha.

In Roman Catholic Liturgy the Akedah (Genesis, xxii, 1–19) is chanted by the priest at the altar on Holy Saturday between the lighting of the Paschal Candle and the Blessing of the Font. It constitutes the third of the twelve lessons called Prophecies. Its chanting is followed by this prayer: 'Oh God the supreme father of the faithful, who throughout the world

[1] James, ii, 21.

[2] Hebrews, xi, 17, 19.

[3] Important references to this subject were made by St. Cyril of Alexandria, St. Athanasius, Ephraim, Ireneus, Isidore of Sevilla, Procopius of Gaza, St. Augustin and Tertullian. Quotations from these references will be given on page 72.

didst multiply the children of they promise . . . and by the paschal mystery dost make Abraham thy servant the father of all nations.'[1]

An allusion to the Akedah is made in a prayer in a canon of the Mass. It is said by the priest when he extends his hands over the consecrated wafer. He prays: 'Upon which do Thou vouchsafe to look . . . and accept them, as Thou didst vouchsafe to accept the gift of Thy just servant Abel and the Sacrifice of our Patriarch Abraham.'

When an altar is consecrated the following Pontifical is said: 'May it (the altar) have as much grace with Thee as that which Abraham, the father of faith, built when about to sacrifice his son as a figure of our redemption.'[2]

The Akedah in Islam. In the third monotheistic religion, in Islam, the Akedah is also of prime importance. This is due to the fact that Mohammed did not intend to found a new religion but to continue the tradition of the faith of Abraham.

The XXXVIIth Sura of the *Koran*[2] is devoted to the Akedah. The Koraņic version differs slightly from the Biblical. This may be due to the absorption of Jewish legendary elements as well as to specific Mohammedan interests.

Abraham (who is called in Arabic, Ibrahim) was asked in a dream to sacrifice Isaac. He at first suspected that the order came from the devil. But when he dreamt the same dream on the following two nights he knew that it originated from God and he decided to carry out the order. The dreams occurred on the eighth, ninth and tenth days of the month of Dhu'l Hidjdja and these days were called the days of 'vision' (of the task demanded), of 'knowledge' (that the order came from God) and of 'the sacrifice' (when Abraham was resolved to carry out the deed).

[1] *The Catholic Encyclopedia*, 1907.
[2] *The Catholic Encyclopedia*, 1907.

The Akedah

Abraham, after his dream, told Isaac bluntly of it and asked him of his attitude. Isaac obediently committed himself to the will of God.

When Abraham was ready to carry out the sacrifice he laid Isaac on his face.

The ram appeared for the vicarious sacrifice from Paradise and was the same animal which Abel offered. This item coincides with a story of the Haggada. In another version the animal of sacrifice was a goat which appeared from Mount Thabir near Mecca. There is an Islamic traditional belief that the horns of the animal sacrificed by Abraham were hung up on the spout of the Caaba in Mecca, a sanctuary which, according to Islamic tradition, was built by Abraham himself. The horns of the ram are believed to have remained on the Caaba until the building was burnt down in the days of Abda'llah Ebn Zoheir.[1]

As regards the place of the attempted sacrifice there are conflicting traditions.

Whilst, according to the oldest tradition, which was expressed by Al-Tha'labi, the son to be sacrificed by Abraham was Isaac, as in the Bible, some Moslem theologians, like Al-Tabari, believed that it was Ishmael, the progenitor of Mohammed.[2] Mohammed is supposed to have said: 'I am the son of the two who were offered in sacrifice.' He meant Ishmael and his father Abd'allah. The latter was due to be sacrificed by his father Abd'almotalleb as thanksgiving to God for the discovery of the well Zemzem but was redeemed by a vicarious sacrifice of a hundred camels.

On the great sacrificial feast Id al-adha, which takes place on the tenth Dhu'l Hidjdja, the Akedah is commemorated in the belief that Ishmael was the son destined for sacrifice. The event is remembered in the takbir of that day, that is a

[1] Al-Beidawi. Quoted from Sale, G.

[2] The Koran.

prayer which expresses the absolute superiority and goodness of the One God.[1]

COMMENTARIES AND LEGENDS ABOUT THE AKEDAH

In order to arrive at an adequate interpretation of the Akedah it is necessary to make use of the exegetical work of Old Testament scholars. Their commentaries in particular are indispensable as they contain most of the historical, geographical, anthropological and other scientific material related to the Akedah.

The purely exegetical work, however, should be supplemented by a study of Talmudic dicta and Jewish legends. To a great extent they are rooted in a tradition which goes back to the dawn of Biblical history.

The Jewish legends can be called the dreams of the people of Israel about their origin and Biblical meaning. From a psychological point of view legends are of special significance. They were created by a process termed in analytical psychology *active imagination*. In the words of G. Adler this process is 'a spontaneous self-development of the original image and not an artificial product intentionally invented'. We may therefore be justified in using the symbols created by legends to illuminate the original Akedah story, provided we are careful to consider the levels on which these symbols were created and operate.

The main findings from the study of commentaries and legends relevant to this work will now be discussed.

Most commentators emphasize the extraordinary character of the story of the twenty-second chapter of Genesis. It is narrated with great simplicity and restraint. The tremendous emotional upheavals of Abraham and Isaac are not directly described but only indirectly referred to.[2] The mini-

[1] Schapiro, M., 1943. [2] Maclaren, A.

mum of bare facts is given and the actual content of the inner experiences of the heroes has to be read between the lines. Every sentence, even every single word is of great significance and so also is everything which remained unsaid but was left to the reader to think out for himself.

Historical Comments. There is no decisive evidence for or against the historicity of the Akedah story. But in the absence of historical documentation a phenomenological study of the story, as told in Genesis, reveals its unique quality. As with every religious phenomenon it is not the general features which are decisive but its specific and unique structure as seen against the background of the general features.

Whether it can or cannot be proved that the Akedah was a historical event the detailed analysis of the story yields a significant clue to the Biblical understanding of man.

An important argument against the historicity of the Akedah might be the existence of similar or parallel stories to the Akedah story. We know from Frazer, Freud and Jung that certain psychological symbols are found in myths of all races and ages and have a universal meaning.[1]

In the study of the similarity of parallel stories the study of their differences, however, must not be overlooked. According to Frankfort[2] these differences might prove to be some-

[1] An example of a parallel story is the Greek legend of the Sacrifice of Iphigenia by her father Agamemnon. As in the case of Isaac, Iphigenia submitted herself obediently to the sacrifice. She was willing to die for the honour of her Mother-land and said that the fall of Troy should be her marriage feast and her monument. In the last moment, however, when Agamemnon turned his head away, Iphigenia was miraculously saved and carried away by the Goddess Artemis who sent a hind for a vicarious sacrifice. (Euripides.)

Another story similar to that of the Akedah is the Indian legend of Cunaçepha. He was the son of a Brahman who intended to sacrifice him in order to please the God Varuna. The gods, however, delivered Cunaçepha and he was adopted by a priest. (M. Müller, *Anc. Sanskr. Lit.* Quoted from Cheyne, T. K., and Sutherland, J., 1914.)

[2] Frankfort, H., *The Frazer Lecture*, 1951.

times more significant than the similarities. The phenomenological study of the Akedah story reveals that it has a unique structure which distinguishes it from the similar extra Biblical stories. Furthermore, it is consistent not only with the religious belief but also with the actual history of Judaism and Christianity.

Geographical Comments. As there is no proof for the historicity of the Akedah story there exists no evidence for the Biblical tradition that the place of the Akedah was the site of the Temple Hill in Jerusalem. It is, however, noteworthy that the distance from Beer-sheba to Moriah, which Abraham, Isaac and the servants may have wandered, is about thirty-eight miles, which is in conformity with a three days' journey. Delitzsch[1] also pointed out that the topography of the Temple Mount was described in Genesis with fidelity.

Of great psychological interest is the symbolic meaning of Mount Moriah. Mount Moriah was, and still is, a tremendous symbol in Biblical religion. In Genesis, xxii, 14 it is related that Abraham called the place 'Jehovah-jireh: as it is said to this day, In the mount of the Lord it shall be seen.' That means that in the future, mankind shall look upon this place in remembrance that there a turning point in the history of the world was reached.

Talmudic tradition excels in symbolic interpretations of the past and the future of Mount Moriah. According to Ber. v.[2] Sem previously had called the place 'Salem' that is the place of 'Peace'. God now united the names given by Sem and Abraham by calling the place 'Jeru-salem'.

The importance attached to the Akedah is further shown by Talmudic legends connecting major events with it. They tell that this is the place where God created Adam, where Adam made the first altar ever built after he was driven out of Paradise, where the altars of Cain and Abel stood and

[1] Delitzsch, F., 1894. [2] Quoted from Beer, B., 1859.

where Noah prayed after his rescue from the flood. Rabbi Simeon[1] pointed out that Abraham did not just build 'an' altar but 'the' altar 'whereon the first ones (of old) had sacrificed'.

After having been the scene of the Akedah, Mount Moriah became the place where 'the Lord appeared unto David' and 'Solomon began to build the house of the Lord at Jerusalem ...'[2] Rabbi Hiyya the Elder and Rabbi Jannai[3] taught that the place of the Akedah became in the time of the Temple the 'Chamber of the Hewn Stone' in the Temple and the spot where 'the Great Sanhedrin sat and sent forth religious teaching to all Israel'. It was the place of instruction (hora'ah), religious awe (yirah) and light for the world (orah).

The role of this most holy place has not yet come to an end but its greatest significance lies in the future. From Mount Moriah, the place of the Akedah, it has been said, the religious rule of the whole world will emanate.[4]

Human Sacrifices. A burnt offering or holocaust consisted in the consumption by fire of the whole body of the victim.[5] The ascent of the flames and smoke symbolically signified the ascent to heaven of the religious intentions of the offerer.[6]

A burnt offering was usually made in times of extreme emergency and often was of extraordinary solemnity. The victim was of pre-eminent value.[7]

The firewood was an essential part of the sacrifice. This is the reason why in verse three of Genesis, xxii, it is mentioned that Abraham 'clave the wood for the burnt offering' and took it with him on the journey.[8]

[1] Quoted from Pirkê de Rabbi Eliezer; by G. Friedlander, 1916.
[2] 2 Chron., iii, 1. [3] *Midrasch Rabbah,* Vayera
[4] Ber. r. and Pesitka. Quoted from Beer, B., 1859.
[5] Exodus, xxix, 18. [6] Linnell, J., 1844.
[7] Hastings, J., 1900. [8] Jacob, B., 1934.

If the victim was a human being his arms and legs were bound. He was laid upon the altar. According to the Koran, Isaac was laid on his face but Jewish tradition related that his eyes were directed towards heaven.

The victim was slain by cutting his throat with a knife. The use of a sword, as can be seen on some pictures of the sacrifice of Isaac, is a western European version. The sixth and tenth verses of Genesis, xxii, describe that Abraham was equipped with a knife. These are the only instances in the Bible in which a knife is mentioned whenever a sacrifice is described.[1] The reason for this is that the reader of the story of the Akedah should not be spared the vivid imagination of the extraordinary horror of the reality of such a sacrifice.

The moral problem arising from Abraham's readiness to sacrifice his son Isaac was a matter of embarrassment for most commentators.

Critics with an anti-Biblical bias used the Akedah chapter in order to attack the ethic of the Bible.[2]

Other theologians attempted to explain and justify Abraham's intention to kill his son by using the argument that Abraham did not believe that he was doing wrong.[3] They also pointed out that Abraham's act can only be understood if one sees him as a man of his time and culture. In ancient Semitic society the father possessed absolute right over the life and death of his children and child sacrifice was therefore a widespread custom, as was mentioned in an earlier chapter.

Although they contain important elements of truth these explanations and justifications need deeper investigation. From the point of view of psychological analysis one should perhaps assume that Abraham suffered from a severe inner

[1] Jacob, B., 1934.

[2] Daumer, Ghillany and others. Quoted from Kamphausen, D. A., 1896.

[3] Dods, M., 1888; Driver, S. R., 1906; Ryle, H. E., 1921.

conflict, the main cause of which was his doubt whether it was really morally right to kill Isaac.

The Personalities of the Story. The significance of the Akedah story is enhanced by the qualities and meanings with which tradition and homiletic speculation endowed the personalities of the story, Abraham, Isaac, Sarah and the two young servants.

Abraham's significance for the whole world is expressed by the saying that God had Abraham in mind when at the beginning of the creation He said: 'Let there be light.'[1] Abraham was called 'the Friend of God'.[2] This is a unique distinction in the whole Bible.

Abraham is considered as the physical and spiritual progenitor of the people of Israel and therefore, in a spiritual sense, of the peoples of New Israel, i.e. the Church. Isaiah[3] expressed Abraham's uniqueness as the father of Biblical religion: 'Look unto Abraham your father, and unto Sarah that bare you: for I called him alone, and blessed him, and increased him.'

As the first of the great patriarchs of the Bible Abraham initiated a new era in the patriarchal order of the world. Until Abraham the father's authority was based on fear. Since Abraham it has been based on love. Love was the principle of the matriarchal order which ruled the world before the patriarchal principle of authority came into being.[4] Abraham, by uniting authority with love, became the creator of the history of Israel.

God said that on the faith of Abraham the world is based.[5] The faith of Abraham was exaltingly praised by the writer of

[1] Genesis, i, 3; according to Ber. r.c. 2, quoted from Beer, B., 1859.
[2] Isaiah, xli, 8, and James, ii, 23.
[3] Isaiah, li, 2.
[4] Bachofen, 1861, quoted from Fromm, E., 1952.
[5] Waijkra r.c., 36, quoted from Beer, B., 1859.

the Epistle to the Hebrews.[1] Abraham was 'the father of faith'.

The high position which Abraham also holds in Islam is shown in the belief that on the day of the resurrection Abraham will take his place, together with Mohammed, by the side of Allah. He will guide the believers into Paradise.[2]

As was expressed in Isaiah,[3] *Sarah* was the great mother of Israel and for that matter of the Church.

Sarah held a unique position amongst all women of Biblical history because she was the only one whom God addressed personally and not through the medium of angels. She was gifted with prophetic vision which was greater than that of Abraham.[4]

In Arabic literature, Sarah, was called the most beautiful woman of her time and her beauty was compared with that of Eve.[5]

Throughout his life *Isaac* was the delight of his parents.[6] His outstanding characteristics were tenderness and absence of aggression. In the Selichoth, the Daily Morning Prayers, he was therefore called 'the tame dove'.[7] He was the first of the great kind ones of Biblical history. Followed by Hosea and Rabbi Hillel his counterpart in the New Testament was Jesus of Nazareth himself.

Isaac gave up his self upon the altar. By doing so he helped to redeem the sins of others.[8] His merits therefore were so great that because of them God will raise the dead in their time.[9]

The tenderness of Isaac's love of his father was shown by some artists by representing him with gentle, almost girlish

[1] Hebrews, xi, 17–19.
[2] Al Tha'labi. Quoted from The Encyclopedia of Islam, 1927.
[3] Isaiah, LI, 2. [4, 5] Quoted from the Jewish Encylcopedia, 1925.
[6] Josephus Flavius. Translated into German by K. Martin, 1852-3.
[7] Asher, D., 1866. [8] 7 Dukes, L., 1842.
[9] Pesitka Rab. Kahana. Quoted from Ryle, H. E., 1921.

features.[1] This points to a 'negative' Oedipus situation of Isaac to Abraham.[2]

Isaac's kindness was equalled by a courage and faith which, at a decisive moment on Mount Moriah, was even greater than that of the father of faith, Abraham.

The two young men whom Abraham took with him on the journey were believed to have been Eliezer and Ishmael.[3] Their role was a very important one for they represented the background of ordinary humanity in the drama. Both Eliezer and Ishmael were distinguished servants but their minds did not grasp the greatness of the situation. Both sensed that Isaac was to be sacrificed and they quarrelled together about which of them would be his heir. A voice from heaven, a Bath Kol, however, told them that neither of them would inherit. When the great moment of the ascent of Moriah arrived they were left behind. 'Abraham said unto his young men, Abide ye here with the ass; and I and the lad will go yonder and worship.'[4]

The figures of the servants show that the drama of Moriah not only has striking similarities with that of Golgotha but with that of Gethsmeane also. For the servants of Abraham remaining at the foot of Mount Moriah are a parallel to the disciples of Jesus. 'Sit ye here, while I go and pray yonder.'[5] The three disciples whom he took further with him fell asleep whilst he worshipped in agony.

The above comments are a random selection of the ideas and fantasies which the luxuriant imagination of the ancients embroidered around the main protagonists of the story. Fanciful as they may seem they give us an indication of the spiritual impact which the Akedah story made on the minds of those who read it.

[1] Tapestry at Halberstadt, Germany. In: Thomson, W. G., 1930.
[2] *See* page 00.
[3] Beer, B., 1859; Pirkê de Eliezer, 1916.
[4] Genesis, xxii, 5.
[5] St. Matthew, xxvi, 36.

The same holds true even of the animals in the story. They too were endowed with extraordinary symbolic significance.

The Animals of the Story. The ass on which Abraham rode was considered to be of special significance. Therefore, Abraham himself, and not his servants, saddled the animal.[1] The ass was created at the dawn of the sixth day of creation which preceded the first Sabbath of the world. It was an ass on which Moses later set his wife and sons when he returned to Egypt.[2] It also was an ass on which the son of David would ride triumphantly as was prophesied by Zechariah.[3]

The ram, like the ass, was created in the twilight of the sixth day of creation because the Akedah was foreseen by God.[4] The ram was grazing under the tree of life refreshing himself from the waters of a nearby stream. When the time of the Akedah arrived an angel brought the ram from Paradise to the thicket of Mount Moriah.

The ram was endowed with the most wonderful features which were described by Pirkê de Eliezer.[5]

The Church Fathers too attributed to the ram the highest symbolic meaning. St. Cyril of Alexandria[6] said that 'the ram represented the figure of a cross'. St. Athanasius[7] wrote that Abraham 'having been restrained from sacrificing Isaac

[1] Beer, B., 1859. [2] Exodus, iv, 20.

[3] Zechariah, ix, 9: 'Rejoice greatly, O daughter of Zion; shout, O, daughter of Jerusalem: behold, thy King cometh unto thee: he is just, and having salvation; lowly, and riding upon an ass, and upon a colt the foal of an ass.'

[4] Aboth. Translated into English by Israelstam, J. In: The Babylonian Talmud.

[5] Pirkê de Eliezer, 1916, quoted Rabbi Chanina ben Dosa who said that on the ashes of the ram the inner altar of the Temple was built. From the sinews the strings of David's harp were made. The skin formed the girdle of Elijah. The left horn was blown on Mount Sinai. But the right horn, which is larger than the left horn, will be blown in the future world that is to come, as was prophesied: 'And it shall come to pass in that day, that the great trumpet shall be blown.' (Isaiah, xxvii, 13.)

[6] St. Cyril of Alexandria, 1881. [7] St. Athanasius, 1844.

saw the Messiah in the ram which was offered up instead as a sacrifice of God'. He commented that the Messiah whom Abraham saw in the ram was the suffering and redeeming Messiah of whom Isaiah prophesied.[1]

Theological Comments. Of all events in Abraham's life the Akedah was held the greatest. The Mishna speaks of ten temptations of Abraham which he had to overcome during his life and of which the greatest was that of the Akedah.

Most commentators see the theological significance of the Akedah in the fact that it represented *the supreme trial of Abraham's faith*[2] and that it was *the triumph of Abraham's faith*'.[3]

The precise nature of the trial, however, always remained a difficulty for the commentators. This was mainly caused by the apparent inconsistency between God's previous promises given to Abraham of eternal salvation through Isaac and God's later command to sacrifice Isaac. What was Abraham to believe?

He might have believed that God only required the surrender of his will to kill but that God would somehow save Isaac.[4] This explanation, however, is unsatisfactory because the will to kill is morally equivalent to the accomplished deed.

Consequently even the greatest theological thinkers remained mystified by the happenings of Abraham's trial. Calvin,[5] e.g. said: 'For as though God were fighting with himself he demands the boy for death. The boy in whom he had before placed the hope of eternal salvation. So this later command was a kind of death of faith.'

[1] Isaiah, liii: 'Surely he hath borne our griefs and carried our sorrows: . . . He is brought as a lamb to the slaughter, and as a sheep before her shearers is dumb, so he openeth not his mouth . . . for the transgression of my people was he stricken . . . and he bare the sin of many, and made intercession for the transgressors.'

[2] Skinner, J., 1912. [3] Dillmann, A., 1897; Ryle, H. E., 1921.

[4] Ryle, H. E., 1921.

[5] Quoted from Ryle, H. E., 1921.

The Akedah

Kierkegaard[1] called the apparent inconsistency of God the 'enormous paradox' of God's command. He now demanded the sacrifice although he previously promised to establish an everlasting covenant with Isaac and Isaac's seed.

As mentioned earlier[2] the very nature of the Akedah story lends itself to *a comparison with the Golgotha story*. There are indeed many striking analogies which were particularly elaborated by the Church Fathers.[3]

[1] Kierkegaard, S., 1939. [2] *See* page 58.

[3] St. Cyril of Alexandria, in his *Third Dialogue of Theodoret*, said that in both events there is a father and only son bearing the material for the sacrifice. Both events happened on the same hill top. The number of days and nights during which both Isaac and Jesus were virtually dead were the same. There also was a subsequent resurrection in both cases.

St. Athanasius of Alexandria, referring to the Epistle to the Hebrews (Hebrews, xi, 17–19), wrote: '. . . and when he (Abraham) was tried, by faith he sacrificed Isaac, and offered up his only begotten son, he who had received the promises. And, in offering his son, he worshipped the Son of God.'

St. Augustine, in *De Civitate Dei*, said, that the thicket in which the ram was caught was a reminder of the crown of thorns which Jesus wore. He pointed out that both Isaac and Jesus carried the wood for their sacrifice up to the mountain of their ordeal, Isaac carrying the firewood and Jesus the wooden cross.

Precopius of Gaza pointed to the similarity of the words of the angel in Genesis with passages of the New Testament. In Genesis, xxii, 16, the angel said to Abraham: '. . . and hast not withheld thy son, thine only son.' In the Gospel of St. John, iii, 16, is written: 'For God so loved the world, that he gave his only begotten Son.' And St. Paul, in Romans, viii, 32, when speaking about the qualities of God, described God as 'He that spared not his own Son, but delivered him up for us all. . . .'

Ireneus said of Abraham: '. . . having with a willing mind yielded up his own only begotten and beloved son as a sacrifice to God, in order that God also might be well pleased, on behalf of his seed, to grant his only begotten and beloved son as a sacrifice with a view to our redemption.' (Quoted from Ryle, H. E., 1921.)

The great similarity of the sacrifice of Isaac and the passion of Christ was expressed by Ambrose in *De Abraham*, I. (Quoted from Smith, A. M., 1922): 'Isaac ergo Christi passuri est typus.' 'Isaac is therefore the prototype of the suffering Christ.'

The Akedah

THE ICONOGRAPHY OF THE AKEDAH

In addition to the homiletic elaboration of the Akedah theme in Jewish and Christian literature there is still another medium of symbolic expression inspired by the Akedah. This is the pictorial representation or the *Iconography* of the sacrifice of Isaac,[1] which is part of Biblical Iconography.

The Iconography of the Akedah affords evidence of how artists throughout the centuries reacted to this particular theme. Pictorial evidence is not used as a rule in Biblical expositions but its value in psychological interpretations is well known and use is therefore made of it in this study.

Artistic creations, it should be pointed out, often resemble dreams and therefore contain unconscious material which is of greatest value for psychological interpretations. The artists who rendered the sacrifice of Isaac have made unique contributions towards the intensification of our imagery of

[1] The story of the Akedah was a frequent topic for artists especially in Europe and the Middle East. The earliest Christian works were found in Roman Catacombs and amongst Asiatic-Hellenistic and Coptic artists. (Smith, A. M., 1922.) An early Jewish rendering of the Akedah, which dates back to the fourth century A.D., was discovered in the recently excavated synagogue of Beth Alpha in Israel. Magnificent Armenian, Arabic, Persian and Turkish works were made especially in the fourteenth and fifteenth centuries by Islamic and Christian painters. (Schapiro, M., 1943.) The greatest masters of European art have made contributions to the subject in the forms of paintings, frescoes, tapestries, stained-glass windows, sculptures, woodcarvings, decorations of lamps, gems, etc.

Artistic representations of the Sacrifice of Isaac can be seen in many English museums, palaces, cathedrals and other places containing art collections. Outstanding works are the tapestry which hangs in the Great Hall of Hampton Court Palace (Law, E., 1927; Marillier, H. C., 1951) and the stained-glass window behind St. Augustine's chair in Canterbury Cathedral. For the purpose of scientific studies, however, the unique collection of photographs, books and periodicals of the Warburg Institute of the University of London is invaluable.

Abraham, Isaac, Sarah, the angel, the servants and of the animals of the story. They have re-created the scenery and atmosphere of the event. They have, for instance, brought to life Abraham's priestly majesty, his terrible weapon, Isaac's gentleness and strength, the angel's grasping of the open blade in the last moment and many other features.

Artists, in their visions, sometimes express ideas or arrive at findings which cannot be obtained from any other source. As is mentioned elsewhere in this study they sometimes have depicted the angel as a woman reminiscent of Sarah. The turning of Abraham's mind was sometimes expressed as a vehement turning of his body away from his victim and towards the heavenly voice. The highest stage of the Akedah drama has been rendered as a common prayer of father and son, after their trial, indicating the commencement of a new era.

Through their particular medium, artists have opened vistas for a deeper understanding of the crucial phase of the drama and its redeeming solution.

The Iconography of the Sacrifice of Isaac was therefore used in this study in order to examine and interpret the unconscious experiences of the artists, in the same way as paintings and drawings are used in psychiatric investigations.

THE OEDIPUS CONFLICT IN THE AKEDAH

The previous chapters on the commentaries and legends dealing with the Akedah were mainly concerned with the presenting of facts about the subject. The following chapters will be devoted to the psychological interpretation of the findings. The first task in this investigation is the study of the Oedipus conflict which must be assumed to have existed between Abraham, Isaac and Sarah.

This does not mean that such a conflict is described in the

Biblical story. All we can say is that the story is remarkable for containing features and details which psychological practice has shown to be symbolic of the unconscious Oedipus situation.

Abraham. At the time of the Akedah Abraham was a very old man.[1] He was at the height of his achievements and it is likely that he felt and feared that his powers as husband and leader of the tribe were now on the decline.

It is interesting to note that, although there is no record in Genesis of Abraham being jealous or afraid of Isaac, these traits of the Oedipus situation were instinctively added by Jewish and Islamic[2] legends.

It was told that the new born babe was so extraordinarily similar in appearance to the father that it was impossible to distinguish one from the other. This story partly had the purpose of proving that Isaac was indeed the son of the centenarian Abraham. But it must also be understood in the light of Frazer's[3] observation which has already been mentioned on p. 20. Similarity of father and son was regarded in primitive society as an alarming sign that the father had died and was born or reincarnated in his son. This meant that the role of the father became endangered and one can assume that Abraham might have felt a similar anxiety as the Hindu fathers whom Frazer described. It is possible that the impulses of Laius were not strange to him nor the desire of King On of Upsala[1] to prolong his life by infanticide.

There are other stories which seem to confirm that Abraham harboured a secret in his heart about which he felt guilty and which he wanted to hide from Sarah. In

[1] According to Genesis, xxi, 5, and Ibn Esra (quoted from Beer, B., 1859) Abraham was probably about hundred and thirteen years old.

[2] Weill, 1846. [3] Frazer, J. G., 1930.

[4] Snorro Sturleson, *The Heimskringla*, 1844.

Genesis it is not mentioned if Abraham told Sarah of his departure with Isaac and the assumption is justified that he left secretly. In the Midrash,[1] however, a farewell is described in which Abraham deliberately hid the truth. He lied to Sarah and told her that he was taking Isaac to the religious School of Sem and Eber, the ancestors of their family. Although this behaviour can also be explained by Abraham's agonizing inner struggle, it points at the same time to an unresolved conflict in him.

As another story suggests, Abraham's Laius Complex towards Isaac was of a particularly tenacious nature. When in the last moment God commanded him not to lay his 'hand upon the lad'[2] he could not fully accept this immediately but wanted to shed at least a little of Isaac's blood.[3] Abraham, in this impulse, wanted to modify the infanticidal act by at least inflicting a vicarious injury to the son as was described by Frazer.[4] But God said further: 'Neither do thou any thing unto him.'[5] This changed Abraham's heart completely and extinguished the last trace of his Laius Complex.

Isaac. There is a legend[6] which indicates that rebellious emotions against his father were not unknown to Isaac. The legend related that Satan came to Isaac and told him that he was the son of a mother deserving pity. His old and demented father was going to slay him. Satan described Sarah in glorious words whilst he spoke about Abraham in a derogatory way. An important detail of the legend is the fact that Satan appeared to Isaac in the disguise of a youth like Isaac himself. This suggests that Satan, as often happens in dream images, was another aspect of Isaac's own personality. The

[1] Jalk. I, 98 nom. *Midrash. B. hajaschar.* Quoted from Beer, B., 1859.
[2] Genesis, xxii, 12.
[3] Hershon, P. I., 1885.
[4] Frazer, J. G., 1930. *See* page 00.
[5] Genesis, xxii, 12.
[6] Tauch. and Jalk., *B. hajaschar. Ber.* r.c. 56. Quoted from Beer, B., 1859.

legend closes with the victorious resistance of Isaac to Satan's accusations. But Beer[1] reports another legend which shows that Satan's visitation did not remain without impression on Isaac.

When the altar was ready for the sacrifice, Isaac implored Abraham to bind his hands and feet firmly, because, so Isaac said, he was a strong youth and Abraham was an old man and he was terrified lest he would instinctively react against the sight of the open blade. According to another version[2] Isaac asked Abraham to bind him because he was afraid in the fear of death to make a reflex movement against the father and even to curse him, thus offending against the precept 'Honour thy father'.[3]

Isaac then went on to say that after his slaughter Abraham should burn him to ashes and place the ashes in Sarah's room. This should be done so that his mother, whenever she would enter her room, would burst into tears and cry: 'Oh this is my son who was slaughtered by his father.' Isaac's hostile impulses against his father and tender feelings for his mother were dramatically expressed in this legend.

Sarah. The legend is told that dreadful foreboding occurred to Sarah when Abraham informed her of the journey which he was to undertake with Isaac. She took Isaac in her tent and kept him there 'all the night and she kissed and embraced him . . . and (in the morning) she said to Abraham: Oh neglect him not.'[4]

The horrible suspicion which can be read in the above words of Sarah became terribly increased when soon afterwards Satan appeared to her. He came in the figure of an

[1] Beer, B., 1859.
[2] Pirkê de Eliezer. Quoted from Friedlander, G., 1916.
[3] Exodus, xx, 12.
[4] Reprinted from *The Legends of the Jews*, by Louis Ginzberg, with the permission of the copyright owner, The Jewish Publication Society of America.

old decrepit man who was an allusion to Abraham. Satan told Sarah of Isaac's agony on the altar of sacrifice and of how he pitifully asked his father for mercy. But Abraham mercilessly slaughtered the son. Sarah was petrified and died from grief.[1]

These stories show that Jewish folklore had the vision of an antagonism of Sarah and Abraham because of her love for Isaac.

The Akedah story describes *the resolution of the Oedipus conflict*. This is achieved to an extent which is never reached in any of the similar stories or legends. In the parallel[2] stories the wish and effort to overcome this conflict we described, but in the Akedah story its complete solution is shown. The resolution of the Oedipus conflict in the Akedah is unique in its completeness because it is brought about by unique religious and psychological phenomena which distinguish the Akedah experience from all other similar experiences. These will be called the *Akedah Motif*.

THE AKEDAH MOTIF I

The *Akedah Motif* is an unconscious constellation of religious-psychological experiences which aim at a complete resolution of parent-child conflicts. It can be called the Biblical experience of the Oedipus Complex. It is characterized by the development of a succession of mental phenomena culminating in a specific kind of super-ego formation. The super-ego of the Akedah Motif is formed by an introjection, moral masochism and instinct transformation which involves the assumption of the existence of an external moral force.

[1] Quoted from Beer, B., 1859.

[2] Like the stories of the sacrifice of Iphigenia and Cunaçepha, which were mentioned on page 63.

The Akedah

It is the purpose of this work to present the phenomena of the Akedah Motif as a new approach to psychiatry.

The Development of the Akedah Motif. The beginnings of the Akedah Motif are as old as the Oedipus Conflict. In the primitive infanticidal era they expressed themselves in the tendencies of the parents to mitigate and modify child murder. In the enlightened Greek and Antique era the Akedah Motif developed into the compromise solution of the Oedipus Complex. These stages can be called primitive and advanced *Akedah tendencies.*

The Akedah Motif was fully developed for the first time in Biblical history by the experiences of Abraham and Isaac. In Abraham it developed as the last and crowning experience which followed a series of extraordinary events of his earlier life. They consisted in the awareness of communications which Abraham felt to be reaching him from an outside power. They are known as *the call of Abraham.* Three times previously in his life he had heard the call of the great external power.[1]

The first time was in Ur when he was sixty years old and the God of Glory appeared unto our father Abraham . . . and said unto him, Get thee out of thy country, and from thy kindred, and come into the land which I shall shew thee.'[2] The second time in Haran, at the age of seventy-five, after the death of his father Terah. This time the call had a promise attached to it. 'Get thee out of thy country, and from thy kindred, and from thy father's house, unto a land that I will shew thee; and I will make of thee a great nation, and I will bless the . . . and in thee shall all families of the earth be blessed.'[3] The third time, the call came to Abraham in Canaan when he was ninety-nine years old. This time God promised that 'Sarah, thy wife, shall bear thee a son . . . and thou shalt call his name Isaac: and I will establish my coven-

[1] Deane, W. J., 1906. [2] Acts, vii, 2, 3. [3] Genesis, xii, 1, 2.

ant with him for an everlasting covenant, and with his seed after him.'[1]

About fourteen years after this last promise God asked Abraham to offer Isaac for a burnt offering. The acceptance of this new communication of God was the first of the *stages of the Akedah experience* proper. It was followed by a period of terrifying thoughts which led to the agony of the deed. It culminated in the transformation of Abraham's mental attitude. Corresponding experiences occurred in Isaac and Sarah. In the language of psychological interpretation these religious experiences can be regarded as experiences of introjection, moral masochism and instinct transformation.

The Phenomenon of Introjection in the Akedah Motif. In the super-ego formation of Abraham the introjection of the mental pictures and moral precepts of his parents and ancestors played a great role. The moral image which formulated Abraham's life most decisively, however, appeared to him as a divine call which came to him from outside.

Some, of course, may prefer to explain the call of Abraham as being due to a *projection* of his own mind, an idea which he produced in himself and believed that it reached him from outside. But even on this assumption the fact remains that the Akedah story expresses the emergence of a specific experience at a particular time and place of Biblical history amongst a particular family, which had unique moral consequences for mankind. The significance of this phenomenon cannot be disregarded even by those who do not share the Biblical attitude. By Biblical attitude is also meant a philosophy which refuses to separate the moral and religious phenomena within from the moral and religious power without.

From this point of view, Abraham not only introjected the mental images of his parents and ancestors but also the con-

[1] Genesis, xvii, 19.

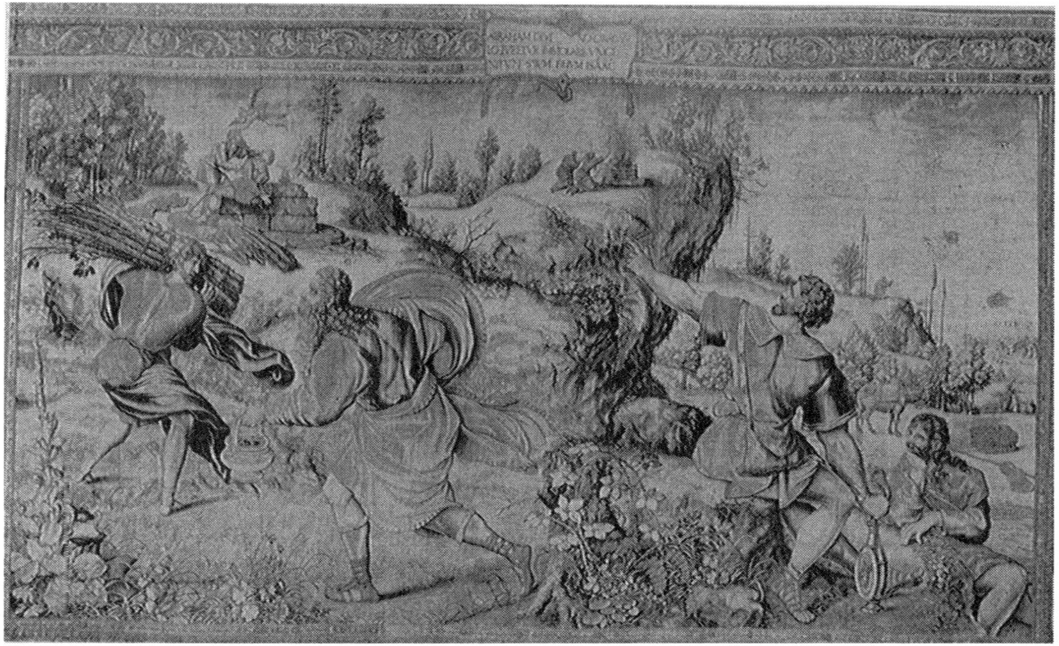

I. Tapestry woven about 1540 by W. Pannemaker. To be seen at Hampton Court Palace. The Sacrifice of Isaac is here shown as a passion of successive stages. The highest stage, in the centre, is the prayer of thanksgiving of Father and son (page 80).

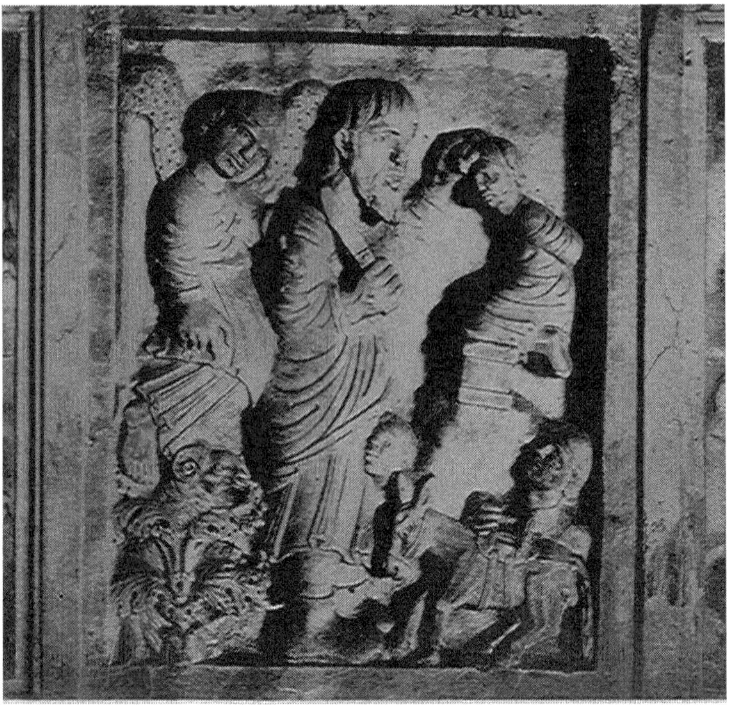

II. Relief on the pulpit at Volterra by Bonusamicus, circa 1200. In this rendering of the Sacrifice of Isaac the figures of Abraham, Isaac and the Angel, who has womanly characteristics, appear to form a family. The sculptor has movingly conveyed a depth of feeling and pious simplicity in the group. At the bottom the two servants, the ass and the ram are seen (page 81).

Kindly lent for reproduction by the Warburg Institute, London University.

tent of the communications of the external divine power. His super-ego was thus decisively formulated by the call of God which he had received before the beginning of his full Akedah experience.

Abraham's Akedah experience commenced with a further audition of God which probably occurred to him during a dream in the night.[1] According to Genesis it began with the words of God: 'Take now thy son . . .'[2] It is of greatest importance to study the wording of this divine communication very carefully because it contains two elements which, although expressed ambiguously, already contain a lead for the solution of the trial.

God continued to say: 'and offer him . . . for a burnt offering . . .'[3] It was noticed by various commentators[4] that God did not say offer him *AS* a burnt offering but *FOR* a burnt offering. This means that God did not explicitly say that Isaac should be slaughtered but rather implied that he merely commanded that Isaac should be brought up to the altar. What was to happen next was left undecided.

God also said: '. . . upon one of the mountains which I will tell thee of'.[5] God did not tell yet on which mountain this was to happen and Skinner drew attention to the fact that it was never imparted in the story where the exact location of the mountain was later given to Abraham. God, by withholding the position of the place, 'put doubt and suspense' in Abraham.[6]

This shows that God's command was not a straightforward one, but was ambiguous from the beginning. It was not a clear order to carry out an act but vaguely implied an order

[1] Pirkê de Rabbi Eliezer, 1916; XXXVIth Sura of the Koran.

[2] Genesis, xxii, 2. [3] Genesis, xxii, 2.

[4] R. Aha in *Midrash Rabba*; Hershon, P. I., 1885; Ibn Esra, *Genesis.* Quoted from Beer, B., 1859.

[5] Genesis, xxii, 2.

[6] R. Huma on the authority of R. Eliezer, *Midrash Rabba.*

to make a choice. Although Abraham 'rose up early in the morning'[1] and set out on his journey immediately, he did not obey the command to kill Isaac simply and blindly as some commentators describe.[2] He began his journey with an agonizing conflict. It was an inner struggle as agonizing and important as the struggle of Jesus when he set out on his way to Gethsemane.

The Moral Masochism in the Akedah Motif. The moral code developed in Abraham's super-ego by his call from God overcame the aggressive and incestuous tendencies of his ego. This state was suddenly altered by the command to sacrifice Isaac. This command emanated from the same source which formerly imposed the powerful repression of aggressive impulses but now it apparently coincided with them. It cruelly allowed Abraham to re-enact his primitive infanticidal wishes but at the same time it forbade him to indulge in them. Abraham is described as being in an acute agonizing state of *moral masochism.* The indications of this in Genesis were taken up and elaborated in legends and commentaries.

Abraham rode for three days to the place of sacrifice. He did not speak during this time, nor did he lift up his eyes.[3] This three days' silent journey stirred the imagination of Kierkegaard[4] who conceived it as a period of terror of thoughts in Abraham's mind.

St. Cyril of Alexandria[5] compared the agony of these three days with the agony of the three days during which Jesus went down to hell before his resurrection. With deep insight into the significance of the martyrdom of the three days Maimonides[6] commented that they were granted to Abraham

[1] Genesis, xxii, 3.
[2] Skinner, J., 1912; Spence, H. D. M., and J. S. Exell, 1897.
[3] Genesis, xxii, 4.
[4] Kierkegaard, S., 1939.
[5] St. Cyril of Alexandria, 1881.
[6] Maimonides. Quoted from Beer, B., 1859.

by God in order to give him time to make his choice. The third day in particular was regarded in Jewish tradition as being of such tremendous importance that it was thought to have happened on the first day of the month of Tischri, on Rosh-Hashana, the New Year's Day, when God will judge everything. According to another version the third day of Abraham's journey coincided with Yom-Kippur, the Day of Atonement.

The ultimate outcome of Abraham's torturing struggle was *unconsciously foreshadowed* by some of his remarks which appear to have been uttered in a sort of trance-like state.

'On the third day Abraham lifted up his eyes, and saw the place afar off.'[1] The meditation of the memorable three days had ended and his mind was set on action. He now knew the exact direction in which to proceed. But he did not yet know what he would find on the summit. He said to his servants: 'Abide ye here with the ass; and I and the lad will go yonder and worship . . .'[2] And then a higher power seemed to direct his further words, which must have shaken him with wonderment when they came forth from his mouth. He continued to say: '. . . and come again to you.' This amazing annunciation was regarded by St. Augustin and Calvin[3] as a sign of Abraham's unconquering faith. Rashi[4] called it an unconscious prophecy. It was, in fact, a sign that after three days of inner struggle Abraham's ascent to a solution had begun.

Whilst ascending the mount, Isaac asked the terrible question: 'Where is the lamb . . . ?[5] And again Abraham spoke with unconscious foreknowledge: 'God will provide himself a lamb . . .'[6] These were the last spoken words recorded in this chapter of Genesis. They were near the summit. The rest of the way they went up in silence.

[1] Genesis, xxii, 4.
[2] Genesis, xxii, 5.
[3] Quoted from Deane, W. J., 1906.
[4] Quoted from Hershon, P. J., 1885.
[5] Genesis, xxii, 7.
[6] Genesis, xxii, 8.

During Abraham's agonizing state of moral masochism his super-ego behaved as if it would wish him to sacrifice Isaac. His present duty seemed to contradict the message and promise of his previous call. He could not understand this dilemma but felt that, in order to understand it later, he had to act now *As If*[1] he was to obey literally. There was no other way than to undergo this ordeal.

During the three days of his journey Abraham unconsciously felt that his ordeal to behave as if he were going to sacrifice Isaac was a fiction which only served to cover a misunderstanding which he was unable to solve. By thoughts he tried to narrow the gap of the misunderstanding to a minimum but he could not bridge it completely.

He could not find the solution as long as he was still in the plain of the desert and not yet on the mount. For the solution could not be found on the level of the plain but on the height of the mountain only. Because, there was no longer thought but deed.

The nearer Abraham came to fulfilling the sacrifice in deed the greater became the mental strain of his as-if experience. But the solution of his conflict could only be achieved by *bearing a maximal strain*. This was an experience which required an extraordinary mental organization. It could not be endured by persons who were made of a weaker mind than that of Abraham. It broke them like a brittle metal is broken—by overstrain.

The mental phenomenon occurring in the mind of Abraham can best be described with the help of a simile taken from the study of metals. There are brittle metals which cannot be overstrained without breaking them and there are ductile metals which can endure overstrain. The ductile metals can be worked to be useful. If the stress applied to

[1] The mental mechanism of the As If has been elaborated by M. Vaihinger, 1924.

such a metal is very large and just less than the breaking stress, then, if the stress is removed, the ultimate strength of the metal, its hardness and elasticity, are tremendously increased. This is the so-called phenomenon of *overstrain.* Abraham, so to speak, was made of ductile metal. He endured the trial of the as-if experience to the utmost. When the stress was removed just at the last moment, Abrahams' strength, vision and love were enormously increased.

In another simile R. Jose C. R. Hanina compared Abraham with a piece of flax of good quality which is beaten by a flax worker. 'The more he beats it the more it improves and the more it glistens: but if it is of inferior quality it cannot give it one knock without splitting it.'[1]

All moral progress comes from personal trial and a superior mental organization of the persons tried. Therefore 'The Lord trieth the righteous: but the wicked and him that loveth violence his soul hateth.'[2] Therefore God tried Job. It is significant that Abraham, in a legend describing the Akedah, was compared with Job. The legend begins with a Prologue in Heaven similar to that in the Book of Job.[3] Satan appears before God, accuses Abraham of wickedness and asks God to try him.[4]

THE AKEDAH MOTIF II

At the Height of the Passion. The Akedah experience consists of a succession of stages of suffering and is in this respect comparable with the passion of Jesus. In fact, many pictorial representations of the Akedah render the story in a succession of scenes reminiscent of the stations of the cross.[5] They show

[1] *Midrasch Rabbah*, Genesis, Vayera.
[2] Psalm, xi, 5.
[3] Job, i, 6–12.
[4] Hershon, P. I., 1885.
[5] This aspect of the Akedah is movingly expressed in a painting by Bronzino which shows six scenes, and in a painting by Israhel van Meckenem which represents five scenes. Photographs of both pictures are in the Warburg Institute, University of London.

Abraham's departure from home, his journey, the scene when he left the servants behind, the ascent of the mount and the altar scene at the height. The last stage of the passion of Abraham and Isaac requires special consideration. It is the deed.

Abraham proceeded from meditation to *deed.* The meditation of the three days was spiritual preparation but the real solution required physical action. Indian and Chinese saints found their apparent solution by meditation only. They did not need deeds because they despised life. Abraham was not content with contemplation only. He believed in the inseparable union of spirit and body. This was the essence of his monotheistic belief in One God only.

Abraham proceeded to the deed. He bound Isaac with his own hands and thrust the knife at Isaac's throat.

At this crucial moment the angel of God intervened.

The urgency of the situation has been dramatically conveyed to us by artists who painted the angel grasping the point of Abraham's weapon, pushing the blade of his sword away or arresting his arm.[1]

A tapestry of the Brussels weaver, W. Pannemaker, which hangs in Hampton Court Palace, shows four way-stations of the passion of the Akedah. (Pl. I.) The first station marks Abraham's and Isaac's fateful departure from the servants who remain, with the ass, at the foot of the mountain, resting, eating and drinking. The second stage is the ascent of Moriah by father and son, Isaac carrying the wood of his own sacrifice on his shoulders as Jesus did on his way to Golgotha, and Abraham carrying a censer as well as the knife. The third station is that of the Akedah. Isaac, bound, lies on the altar; Abraham, at the height of his agony is almost ready to carry out the sacrifice when at the last moment the angel of Jehovah intervenes. But the last and highest station is not that of the averted sacrifice. It is that of the sacrifice of the ram and of the common prayer of thanksgiving of father and son, which stands for the beginning of a new era.

[1] This is demonstrated in paintings by Giovanni Antonio Bazzi and Luca Giordano and in a Religious Icon to be found in the British Museum which is reproduced in Pl. III. Photographs of the paintings are in the collection of the Warburg Institute, London University.

The Akedah

In the Iconography of the Akedah the saving angel is often painted as a female figure of beauty.[1] This is of psychological interest as the Bible only knows male angels.

A remarkable representation of the angel was made by Bonusamicus. In his relief on the pulpit at Volterra a woman with wings stands behind Abraham, forming with Isaac a family group (see Pl. II).[2]

According to psychological interpretation the female figure of the angel would have to be taken as a symbolic image of Sarah. And indeed, the thought is justified that Sarah's influence arrested the blade, brought the ram, and stood by Abraham's and Isaac's side in the moment of their greatest need.

This is also suggested by the Haggadic sources. There it is stated that Sarah had more prophetic vision than Abraham. She must have influenced him deeply throughout their lives. The last words which she said to Abraham before he went on the journey with Isaac must have especially affected him during the three days of meditation and must have reverberated in his mind during the agony of the last moment: 'Oh . . . I pray thee, take heed of thy son and place thine eyes over him.'[3]

It is therefore psychologically not incorrect to say that the angel spoke with the voice of Sarah. But Sarah was only the mediator and not the real power of the new command. Abraham did not accept the command of a mediator and

[1] This, for instance, is shown in the above-mentioned painting by Giovanni Antonio Bazzi. A significant version of the angel was painted by P. Testa. In his work a number of female angels are seen, one of them, carrying in great haste the ram in her arms, the vicarious sarifice. This version is very rare in Western art but, as Schapiro, M. (1943) pointed out, common in Islamic art.

[2] The setting of a family is also given in an Alexandric-Coptic fresco at El Bagawat. It shows a woman without wings standing by the side of Abraham and Isaac.

[3] *The Legends of the Jews*, Louis Ginzberg (1908).

insisted that God Himself should speak to him.[1] Therefore 'the angel of the Lord called unto Abraham out of heaven the second time, and said, By myself have I sworn, saith the Lord . . .'[2] This means that God did comply with Abraham's invocation and spoke Himself to him. This oath of God was the only one recorded in the history of the patriarchs.[3] It is 'a point of unprecendented lustre in the Old Testament: for Jehovah here swears what he promises, as he does nowhere in his intercourse with the patriarchs.'[4]

Abraham did not lay his hands upon Isaac. The gap was filled. The solution was found. The tendencies of thousands of years had reached fulfillment. A fundamental change had taken place in Abraham, *a turning of mind* which divided the history of the world into two parts: one before and one after the Akedah.

The turning of Abraham's mind was symbolically expressed in artistic works by the turning of Abraham's body. In a Religious Icon from a French Bible (in the British Museum) Abraham's head was turned almost a hundred and eighty degrees towards the heavenly messenger (see Pl. III).[5]

When Abraham turned towards the calling angel he was so struck because he recognized the voice. He had heard it calling him three times before in his life. His turning was a returning to his calling.

The Instinct Modifications in the Akedah Motif. Through the experience of the turning Abraham's instincts underwent a decisive modification. During this process, phenomena occurred which were characteristic of the Akedah Motif and were not encountered in similar experiences of super-ego

[1] Hershon, P. I., 1885. [2] Genesis, xxii, 15, 16.

[3] Jacobs, B., 1934. [4] Delitzsch, F., 1894.

[5] Mitellus (after a Titian painting in Santa Maria della Saluta, Venice) represented Abraham at the moment when the angel called from heaven. His whole body is struck as by lightning, twisted and turned vehemently away from the place of sacrifice and towards the calling angel.

formation. They concerned the promotion and modification of the life instinct.

A fundamental effect of Abraham's change of outlook was the realization that God demanded life and not death. Abraham realized that the meaning of the commanded sacrifice was not to kill his son but to dedicate his son's life for lifelong service to God. He completely rejected the former dominance of his death instinct and entirely abandoned his aggressive tendencies against Isaac. His life instinct was tremendously promoted and with it a new love emerged in him for Isaac which became the crowning experience of his religion.

The idea of renewed life is represented symbolically by a surprising detail on the Alexandric-Coptic fresco referred to earlier.[1]

Intimately connected with the promotion of his life instinct was the promotion of a vital *need* in Abraham *to act.* By his resolute action he actually gained the victory of his life instinct over his death instinct. The desire to act and its counterpart, the need to meditate, are fundamental religious attitudes. It was a significant effect of the Akedah experience to strengthen the desire to act. It taught that meditation, or faith alone, is not sufficient but that action too is essential in Biblical religion. This is what was meant by James[2] when he said: 'Was not Abraham our father justified by works, when he had offered Isaac his son upon the altar. . .? Ye see then how that by works a man is justified, and not by faith only.'

The most important effect of the strengthening of Abraham's life instinct was the *increase of his object love.* This was a

[1] It shows Isaac holding a small box in his hands and Sarah with a similar box. A box, in the language of symbolism, is a container like a uterus. A uterus contains new life. It seems as if the artist's unconscious vision has seen one of the deepest meanings of the Akedah.

[2] James, ii, 21 and 24.

process which can best be interpreted satisfactorily in the light of Biblical religion.

According to psycho-analytical theory, introjected parent and other images become ego-ideals and the aim of self-love or secondary narcissism. By this process, object-love which was formerly directed to the parents and other persons is withdrawn. A different aspect is gained if the Biblical view is accepted that Abraham's most formative image of his super-ego was the introjected call of God. According to this view he directed libidinous energy to the ego-ideal of his call, which had two consequences.

Abraham loved the call as something which was now in him, and thus part of himself. He loved the call with narcissistic or self-love. Whatever the call demanded was experienced in relation to his self-love. The command to sacrifice Isaac could be rationalized as being the opportunity to prove the greatness of his self-righteousness and could be justified because of reasons of self-preservation. By meditating about this his self-love increased and almost drove him to infanticide.

But Abraham's love for the ego-ideal of his call, which contained an altruistic aim, also had another and far more important consequence. It amplified his object-love by decreasing his self-love. This tendency clashed with the first-mentioned tendency contributing to the agony of Abraham's moral masochism, but, in the last moment, gained complete victory.

The amplification of Abraham's object-love was directed to Isaac in the first place but embraced all human beings and, because of the promise attached to the call, even future generations. It was a love which aimed at the happiness of all mankind in a purified and redeemed world. This mental attitude is *messianic love.* It became the most dynamic moral power of Judaism and Christianity with widespread cultural effects.

The Akedah

The unique manner of the emergence and the unique qualities and effects of messianic love justify the assumption of the intervention of a moral power outside man which was introjected into man. This external moral power we are accustomed to call God.

The Change of the Name of God. The decisive change in Abraham's spiritual attitude is illustrated by the change of the Divine name in the Akedah story. God, at the beginning of the story, is called *Elohim* but at its end He is called *Jehovah.*[1]

The interpretation of the great significance of the change of the name of God in Genesis xxii follows Jacob.[2] He was of the opinion that Elohim, who tempted Abraham, was only a servant of God and not the real God Himself. Abraham also obeyed the servant of God, but he did so with a mental reservation. The open blade in the last moment of his ordeal brought about the change. He heard God's real voice and no longer obeyed the inferior Elohim but God Himself. He exchanged the Elohim for Him. And therefore 'Abraham called the name of that place Jehovah-jireh',[3] because he saw Him on the mount, the Holy Hill of the psalm.[4]

In the light of this interpretation Abraham's vision of the very nature of God underwent a change after the turning phase of the Akedah experience. According to his comprehension Elohim's command to sacrifice Isaac was not inconsistent with God's nature. Elohim, in this respect, represented

[1] As is generally known, the use of these different names of God in Genesis is held to be due to different sources. Such a theory need not be inconsistent with the Jewish tradition that Moses was the compiler of Genesis, and it may be noted that the more general name, Elohim, is used particularly when the patriarchs are in contact with the pagan peoples, while Jehovah belongs particularly to God as He reveals Himself and His character to Abraham and others. This difference can be felt in the rendering of the Authorized Version of the Bible, where Elohim is simply translated God, while Jehovah is THE LORD.

[2] Jacob, B., 1934. [3] Genesis, xxii, 14. [4] Psalm xxiv, 3 ff.

the non-Biblical belief that destruction ultimately is as justified as creation. This belief is derived from the opinion that the world is governed by an eternal cycle of birth and death and that to obey God means to resign to the rule of this circular movement. Life itself has no intrinsic value because our goal is to submerge in the harmony of the eternal circular movement. Love to any particular person is therefore not specially valued in this belief. This provides a justification for infanticide. It is, in fact, a perfect rationalization for the death wish of the Laius-Oedipus Complex.

But this was only one aspect of the Elohim. In the ambiguous wording of his command he made mental reservations as to the moral value of infanticide which laid the foundation of Abraham's change of mind.[1] Elohim, if rightly understood, already spoke with the voice of Jehovah.

Jehovah commanded sanctification of life. This meant that the works done *here and now* are essential for the world to come.

Jehovah commanded personal love to definite persons as the highest expression of the intimidation of the Divine Love. Therefore infanticide must be abolished and also the compromise solution of satisfying one's hatred by vicarious acts. A new love must be kindled in the heart of man. This was Abraham's vision on Mount Moriah.

The Aspects of the Akedah Motif. The Akedah Motif concerns the moral development of family life. It consists of the aspects or motifs of the father, son, mother and daughter. The motifs of parents and children, reacting on each other, form the Akedah Motif of the family.

The outstanding phenomenon of the *Abraham Motif* is the initiative of the father in overcoming the family conflict. By his struggle, agony and practical example Abraham gave the

[1] *See* the remarks on p. oo.

lead for the resolution not only of his Laius Complex but also of the Oedipus Complex of Isaac and the Jocasta Complex of Sarah.

His initiative made him the central figure of the Akedah drama. This point is impressively illustrated in many works of art. Abraham was often represented as a Lord and priest, wearing flowing white draperies and sometimes having a halo.[1] In order to show his power Abraham frequently holds a terrible sword of enormous proportions.[2] Abraham had the right and the power to use the sword but he did not use it. He did what his descendent Malachi later proclaimed to be the first requirement for the coming of the messianic age, he turned his heart to his child so that the heart of his child turned to him. Abraham was frequently called 'the father of faith' but he should also be called 'the father of love', because it was through love of his son that he ascended to the Akedah.

A moving aspect of Abraham's love of Isaac was shown by Rembrandt's paintings 'The Sacrifice of Abraham' and 'The Return of the Prodigal Son'.[3] They reveal that Abraham's love of his son was the love of a father for his prodigal son. All sons in their Oedipus aggression are prodigal sons and we can assume that Isaac, before the Akedah, was no exception to this. In the two paintings, the sons are naked as a child is when he is born, thus indicating that they were born again. In both pictures the sons' faces cannot be seen. They are

[1] An example is a tapestry at Halberstadt in Germany which was woven in the twelfth century. (Thomson, W. G., 1930.)

[2] This is, for instance, seen in a stained-glass window in Canterbury Cathedral which dates from *circa* 1230 and is situated behind St. Augustin's Chair. It is also seen in a painting by a follower of Toriti in the Chiesa Superiori di S. Francesco, Assisi.

[3] 'The Sacrifice of Isaac' was painted in 1635. 'The Return of the Prodigal Son' was finished in 1663, shortly before Rembrandt's death. It is one of the most stirring and monumental works of this great painter. Both paintings are in 'The Hermitage' in Leningrad. (Bodkin, T., 1948.)

blotted out; in the first case by the father's hand and in the second by his clothing. The fathers' faces in both pictures are shown with an expression as if shining in supernatural joy. Although the second picture was made twenty-eight years after the first one, the fathers appear to have a similar face.

The main developmental stages in the Abraham Motif were the experiences of the temptation and the turning. When the Elohim tempted Abraham he wished to prove to God his self-righteousness by obeying the terrible command and to give up his messianic tasks which he had obtained through previous calls. The stage of temptation is the phase of moral masochism. Ego and secondary narcissism are for infanticide. Super-ego and the awareness of the messianic call decide against it. The stage of the turning is characterized by the introjection of a further call of God and the father's ultimate choice to conquer his Laius Complex completely.

When, as an Infant, Isaac reverently introjected the image of his father he also introjected the experience of his father's call of God. But as Abraham was tempted to interpret his calling as a justification to prove his self-righteousness by committing infanticide, so was Isaac tempted to use his introjected ideal as a justification for harbouring patricidal ideas against the 'father tyrant'.

During their three days' journey not only Abraham but also Isaac must have been tortured by intense moral masochism. Father and son fought the same battle. On the one hand Isaac behaved as if he were obediently following his father's command but on the other hand he considered if it were not better to kill his father before he was killed by him.

But at the height of his agony Isaac completely conquered

his Oedipus hatred. When Abraham in the last moment looked into the eyes of Isaac[1] he was amazed and finally changed by what he saw. 'The eyes of Isaac looked towards the angels on high, and Isaac beheld them, but Abraham saw them not.' Isaac saw Heaven because he had overcome his Oedipus Complex completely. But Abraham saw it not for he still struggled with the last convulsions of his Laius Complex. Although Abraham had taken the initiative to resolve the Laius-Oedipus conflict completely it was Isaac who succeeded first in doing so. In this respect Isaac was greater than Abraham. By the surrender to the father's command *the son is greater than the father.*

Isaac, so the legend tells, died in the moment of his final surrender. But during the moment when Abraham looked into the eyes of Isaac he gained his last strength to resolve the last traces of his Laius Complex. The soul of Isaac returned into his body. Father and son had saved each other.

Elaborating the text of the Akedah chapter psychologically one might perhaps say that, although *Sarah* does not appear personally in the story, her influence in its course is so great that it decides the issue.

Sarah's central experience was her experience of Abraham's call of God. This destined her to overcome her Jocasta Complex completely. She unconsciously felt what the purpose of Abraham's journey was and was tempted to prevent Isaac from following his father. By letting Isaac go she conquered her Jocasta Complex.

But her undivided love for husband and son accompanied both in their final, bitter struggle, protected and saved them. The love of Sarah was with Abraham and Isaac during the three days of the journey. It influenced Abraham when he spoke to the servants and to Isaac during the ascent of the

[1] Targum of Palestine. Quoted from Ryle, H. E., 1921.

mount. It stayed his arm in the last moment. Sarah was the angel.

Sarah was the moving force of the Akedah. Her love was greater than that of father and son. She was the mother.

The Akedah story, as the Oedipus story, does not contain a daughter figure. But the idea of the Akedah Motif, as that of the Oedipus Complex, includes a daughter experience. In the Oedipus Complex the daughter's hatred of her mother was called the Electra Complex. This term was derived from the Agamemnon-Clytemnestra myth. The daughter aspect of the Akedah Motif is characterized by the complete abandonment of the Electra Complex. An outstanding Biblical example of such an experience is given in the Book of Ruth.

Ruth, the Moabite, gained this experience by her love of her mother-in-law Naomi, through which she was converted to the belief of Abraham. So great was Ruth's contribution to the raising of the moral standard of family life that she was deemed worthy of becoming the ancestress even of King David, and through his line, of Jesus of Nazareth.

The Akedah story itself does not give a clear indication of what follows. One can, however, draw the conclusion that it marked the beginning of a new relationship between father and son which initiated a new era in the family relationships of man.

Its realization depends on a situation in which selfish aims are abandoned and real personal love and dedication to God's call are possible.

From the phenomenological point of view this new relationship can be described as *a covenant between parent and child* which inaugurated a new era of moral code. A pictorial representation of the foundation of the new covenant is seen in the tapestry at Hampton Court. (Plate I.) The last and

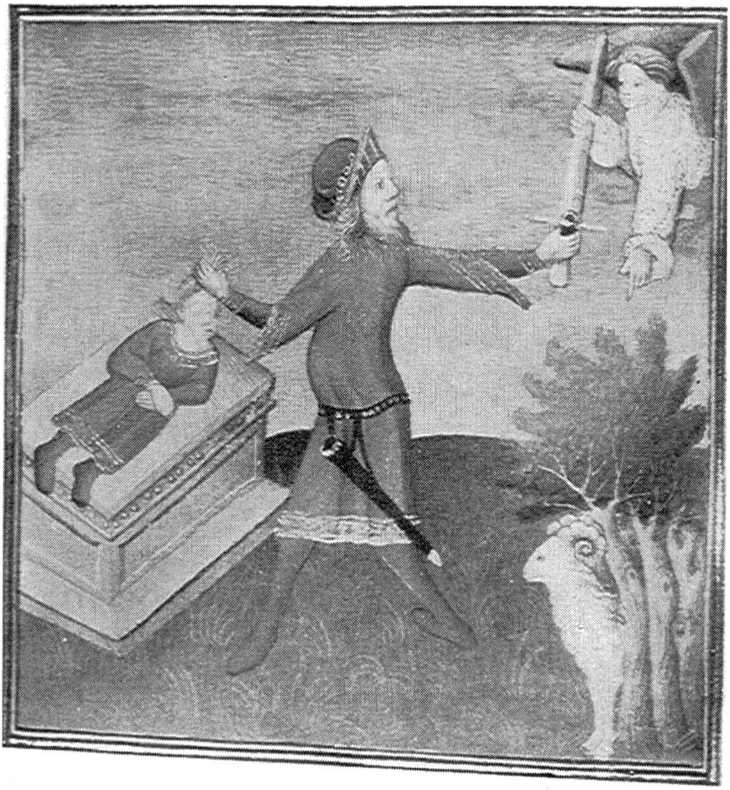

III. Religious Icon from a French Bible, fifteenth century. Photograph at the Warburg Institute. Here the turning of Abraham has been dramatically depicted. At the last moment Abraham, whilst still in a position to make the sacrifice, has turned his head completely to face the angel. The angel is female and grasps the blade of the large sword. She points to the ram which stands in dedicated submissiveness (page 96).

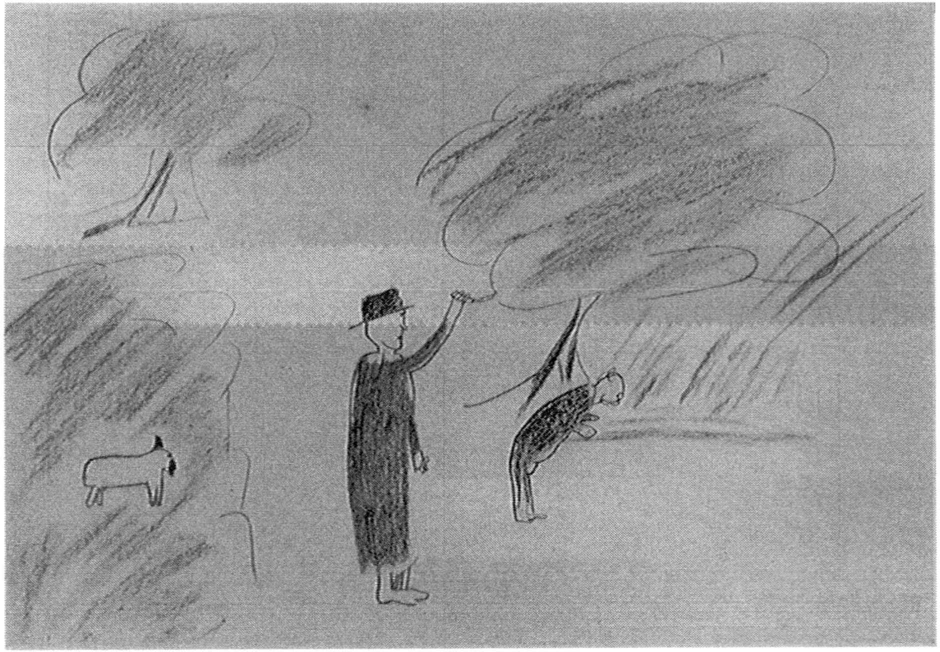

IV. In this crayon-drawing of a boy of fourteen, attending a Child Guidance Clinic, Isaac is shown bowing submissively to Abraham's task. The ram too has a submissive stance (page 97).

highest stage in the passion of the Akedah, which this tapestry shows, is the prayer of thanksgiving of Abraham and Isaac. On the top of the summit they kneel in front of the altar in great emotion. They inaugurate the new covenant.

CLINICAL OBSERVATIONS OF THE AKEDAH MOTIF

The Akedah Motif is not only a theoretically important religious phenomenon. It has, above all, great practical and clinical importance because it is experienced in all human beings.

The clinical observation of the Akedah Motif, however, often requires a particular approach. The reason for this is that religious experiences, like sexual experiences, often do not lie on the surface of consciousness but in the unconscious layers of the mind. They also need special methods for their recognition.

When the Oedipus Complex was postulated, most psychiatrists and the majority of the lay public at first rejected its sexual implications. Whilst this resistance, through the results of analytical work, has now been largely overcome, another resistance against psychological facts has become apparent: the resistance against religious matters. In a similar way in which sex used to be taboo, religious belief is now taboo amongst wide circles of psychiatrists in the lay world. The taboo against the serious admission of religious experiences is even more severe than the taboo against sexual matters used to be and is more difficult to overcome.

The essential prerequisite for the recognition of the reality of religious experiences in others is the experience of this reality in one's self. The main way to arrive at it is through prayer. Prayer in the recognition of religious experiences plays an equally important role as dreams do in the interpretation of sexual experiences. Few people consciously pray but there is hardly a person who, unconsciously, has not prayer-like experiences. By this is meant experiencing as-if a power outside and above man personally and morally influenced him.

If seen in this light many observations of psychological experiences assume religious significance even if they were not consciously experienced as being of a religious nature.

Patients suffering from problems deriving from their Akedah experience are usually seen by psychiatrists in the stage referred to as moral masochism, because this is the stage in which clinical signs and symptoms are most apparent. This inner struggle is in fact a religious one as was that of Abraham and Isaac. The therapeutic solution is the turning to the principle of selfless love, an experience akin to religious conversion.

In clinical practice well-known phenomena of parent-child conflicts may gain new significance if they are interpreted in the light of the Akedah Motif. Mechanisms of the Laius-Oedipus Complexes undoubtedly play a part, but examination of the phenomena may sometimes reveal a succession of details which strikingly resemble experiences characteristic for the Akedah Motif.

Fathers, for instance, can be observed who change their previous apparent loving attitude towards their sons and seriously turn against them. This change, although possibly in preparation for a long time, may occur suddenly, together with an urge for action which seems to be dictated by a moral power. The moral quality of this power may become particularly obvious if the son's behaviour arouses the father's demand for punishment, as in the case of a teacher whose son falls short in his scholastic achievements or of a preacher who discovers that his son has misbehaved sexually.

The father may then turn against his son with a severity which is out of proportion to his son's actual misbehaviour. He attacks him in righteous indignation and with the conviction that he is directed to do so by the highest moral law. But closer observation may reveal that he does so with a heavy heart and that he is at least as much, if not more, distressed about his own attitude against his son as about his son's failure. He may unconsciously be aware that his son's misbehaviour is only a pretext for the unleashing of his own Laius Complex which he wishes to overcome but at the same time he is bewildered about the apparently moral call in him which orders him to be severe with his son. He is in a state of moral masochism.

During treatment it may become apparent that a father's distress becomes more agonizing the more he continues in his severity against his son, but that during this process he also comes nearer to the solution of his problem. There may come a moment during therapy when another change occurs in the father's mind and he turns to his child in love. Often the mother's influence, directly or indirectly, plays a great role. The turning of the father's mind may be indicated by a decision showing that he took the initiative in the resolution of the conflict. But the final result will depend on his son's reaction. The father's change of mind is sometimes accompanied by a feeling of sudden new insight and intense happiness as has been described in experiences of religious conversion. The role of therapy is to unravel the Laius and Oedipus Complexes and to suggest that their full resolution can only be brought about by selfless love. Practical ways of showing such a love should be suggested and in suitable cases the use of prayer may be advised.

In the clinical observation of these processes the study of *Akedah dreams* is often of great value. Here, in the first place, boys' nightmares of their fathers' aggression should be mentioned. The role which the Oedipus and Castration Complexes play in these dreams is, of course, well known. It is also generally known that the aggressive father figure often holds a knife in his outstretched hand which, psychoanalytically, usually is interpreted as a dangerous phallic symbol. It may, however, not be unjustified to consider the possibility that the dream symbol of the threatening knife may also be a symbol of the sacrificial knife of the father with infanticidal tendency.

An unusually vivid and instructive Akedah dream was recorded by Edmond Gosse in the narrative of his early life, entitled 'Father and Son'.[1] Following an incident of rebellion against his revered father, the nine-years-old Edmund dreamt that he was madly galloping through infinity, hurried on by an overwhelming force. He was utterly helpless as he was *bound hand and foot* like Mazeppa.[2] It seemed to him as if an immense force were driving him on to reach a vital goal, but much as he craved to reach it he felt that he would never succeed. He could just see the goal in the far distance: it consisted of ruby-coloured letters of the word *carmine*. As regards the significance of this word Edmund Gosse explained that his father used to produce water-colour paintings and that the most precious of his father's paints was an intense crimson, which was the only one Edmund was forbidden to use. Carmine therefore became for him the symbol for all he desired most.

This dream tragically reveals the agonizing conflict between father and son. His father, not unlike the revenging husband who punished Mazeppa, as an overpowering force, drove him into the wilderness of emotional conflict. Although it is not explicitly stated in the dream one can perhaps imagine the father in the symbolic figure of a galloping, wild horse,

[1] Gosse, E., 1907.

[2] Koledinsky Ivan Stepanovich Mazeppa (1644?–1709) was a famous leader of the Cossacks. In his youth he had an affair with a married woman and, as a punishment, was tied naked to the back of a wild horse by her husband and driven into the lonely steppe where he was meant to die. (R. Nisbet Bain, 1905.)

as this is frequently a terrifying father symbol in night-mares.

The force of the father bound him hand and foot. In this symbolic description, the Akedah situation is expressed in rare clearness. Both, the force and the boy were feverishly pushing on towards a goal, and their salvation depended on reaching it. The goal was *carmine*, that is the treasure of his father, which may have symbolized his father's high moral calling. But a despair in Edmund's heart told him that his father and he could never reach the goal. This completely illustrated the actual life situation of Edmund and his father, which tragically never changed substantially in their lives. His father, a man of outstanding moral qualities, still remained captivated by self-righteousness and never reached the stage of real selfless love for his only son. And Edmund, in spite of being no less distinguished than his father, by noblest aspirations, remained rebellious against his father's ideals until the end. Both had valid reasons for their aggression and spiritual fight against each other but in the depth of their hearts the Laius and Oedipus Complex was never resolved and true selfless love could not unite them.

Another revealing approach in the clinical observation of the Akedah Motif is the study of *paintings of patients*. The present writer mainly studied paintings of children attending a Child Guidance Clinic. Some of these paintings illustrate dreams which unconsciously show features of the Akedah Motif.

A thirteen-years-old boy, for example, told that he had a terrifying dream of a horse chasing and trampling him. A horse, in dream symbolism, often represents the father. A sketch of the dream showed a fierce horse, standing up and trampling on the figure of a boy. The boy was lying on the ground, outstretched and immobile in a completely passive position which appeared to be inappropriate to his dangerous situation. This boy felt threatened by his father's moral precepts. He suffered, but submitted himself to his father's demands.

Other relevant paintings are illustrations of the Akedah story which were produced after the Akedah chapter was read to the children. These pictures, so to speak, represent a *Clinical Iconography* of the Akedah Motif.

A boy, aged fourteen, carefully illustrated the Akedah story by painting Abraham building an elaborate altar with Isaac conspicuous by his absence. When asked where Isaac was he said indignantly that he was not there because he did not wish to look on and watch how the altar on which he was soon to die was made. He was doing something else during the short time he still had to live. The lad was very immature and not only symbolically ran away from his duties towards his father and teachers but also actually ran away from school, truanting so excessively that he had to be excluded from school.

Another fourteen-years-old boy was referred to the Clinic because of attacks of panic during which he felt that everything was going far away. When asked to make an illustration of the Sacrifice of Isaac he produced a striking picture. It showed Isaac having made the fire for his sacrifice and deeply bowing, whilst Abraham's hand is stretched out to slay him. (see Pl. 4). It is interesting that the boy's and the ram's submissive stance and face are drawn in similar curves. This boy suffered from an intense Oedipus conflict which caused his terrifying attacks. His readiness to submit to his father, which was indicated in the picture, proved to be the decisive factor in his treatment.

The clinical significance of the Akedah Motif is best illustrated by a *case history*. The case history which is given describes a problem not infrequently found at Child Guidance Clinics.

Peter, a seven-years-old boy, was referred by the School

Doctor because of increasing dreaminess, preoccupation, and destructive behaviour. This reached a peak when he laid waste a garden, emptying a pond and killing the fish. At home he was off his food, was extremely restless and would sometimes hit his mother.

Peter's father is a store-keeper. The marriage of the parents was quite happy till the father returned from the War. Since then the father exercised an almost military discipline over the home, bullying Peter and his twenty-two-years-old brother Robert, and keeping the mother short of money. He would not allow the mother to punish Peter but beat him himself during his frequent attacks of depression and bad temper. When advice was offered to him by his doctor and a marriage guidance counsellor he was not receptive and did his best to ensure that his wife had no contact with authorities. He also had refused to attend a Child Guidance Clinic on behalf of Peter.

Peter's Headmistress commented that the boy was very polite and that his relationships in school were good but that he had a tendency to go wild at times. The Headmistress's relations with Peter's mother were cordial but his father was unknown to the school. She had known the mother for several years and noticed that the strain of the marital discord was telling on her.

At the clinical interview Peter was found to be physically healthy and well developed. He had brightly-shining, grey eyes which sometimes gleamed sadly, and a comely, almost girlish face.

His intelligence on the Terman-Merrill Scale ranked as high average, his successes on this test showing a normal scatter.

In his behaviour he was hyperkinetic and flighty, continuously moving about the playroom from one toy to another, as if he wanted to overcome an inner tension by over-activity.

He also was extremely talkative. There were frequent boastful but also apologetic references to fighting: 'I'd like to be a boxer. . . . The boys keep getting on at me and say that I'm the one who starts it, but I'm not.'

Frequently he mentioned his father and it was quite obvious that he was strongly influenced by his personality. '. . . and my Daddy has big books, they cost a lot of money . . . he gives me the cane . . . he also combs my hair . . . he hits my Mummy, I often see it . . .' He added: '. . . and I hit Mummy, this is very naughty of me. . . . Oh! Mummy and Daddy often have rows.'

There was no doubt that Peter suffered severely from the frequent scenes between his parents. In his despair he imitated their destructive behaviour and it is not unjustified to assume that his behaviour towards the pond and fish was a symbolic expression of this. A pond is a common unconscious female and mother symbol and fish a common male and father symbol.

An outstanding feature of Peter's personality was, that, against expectation, he did not show hatred of his father. On the contrary, he recounted his caning and the bad treatment of his mother sadly, but otherwise revealed a submissive and tender love for his father. From his remarks about his mother he showed that he was also devoted to her.

When the mother made her statement she broke down with emotion. She appeared to be beside herself, a heart-broken, worn-out woman who eased her troubled mind by violent outcries and tears.

'My husband has been a good father . . . he must be ill . . . he can be very sweet . . . he does not drink, has no vices . . . his life is in the home. . . . We were happy before.

'It all started when he came back after the War. He is like a Sergeant-Major. He says that I don't obey and have therefore broken the marriage law. . . . He says that I have turned our sons against him . . . he is madly jealous of the sons . . . but, please believe me, I have always taught them to love their father and to do as they are told.

'He says that I have given him a life of hell . . . he calls me bad and wicked . . . perhaps, there is something wicked in me. . . . I try to pray to God.

'When I put Peter to bed recently, he said: "I wish Daddy loved you, I wish you were both happy, then I'd be happy too."

'One year ago it became unbearable and since then I wish I could have a separation. A year ago my husband turned Robert out of the house, our elder son. It was a dreadful scene. One evening Robert watched television. His father told him to leave the room. The boy showed spirit and his father went at him in a terrible rage as if he were killing him. I threw myself between them.'

From the mother's statement, the conclusion could be drawn that a critical Oedipus conflict existed in the family. As often happened during the War when the husband was away and the mother lived alone with her children it was likely that also in this case the mother became over-attached to her sons. She developed an intense Jocasta Complex, especially towards Robert, the elder son. She made, however, some positive remarks about her husband which gave rise to some hope for her treatment.

It was obvious that no full picture of the marital situation could be gained without seeing the father too.

A sympathetically worded invitation was sent to the father in which an appeal was made to him to assist the Clinic in helping Peter. The father came.

He had the same grey eyes as Peter but they had a penetrating and aggressive look. His facial expression revealed intense worry and suffering. He was a simple, uneducated man, spoke slowly and had difficulty in thinking and expressing himself. He appeared to be a person of deep feelings and high principles.

He said: 'I loved them all . . . I put my life in my family . . . but what results! . . . Peter is now the only one I have got . . .'

He had very strict ideas about what is right and wrong and his ethics centred around discipline and doing what one is told. These ideas he linked with his belief in God, the Church, law and order. No doubt, his service in the Army had reinforced this belief which had grown in him to an obsessional idea of duty and obedience. It was this standard with which he judged the family situation on his return.

When he found his wife and sons rallied against him he developed an intense Laius Complex, feeling it a high duty to his principles of conduct to punish his family severely, but especially Robert, the elder son.

He told the story of his conflict with Robert in bitter and highly excited terms and it became apparent that this was the conflict which tortured him most.

'Robert,' he said in a trembling voice, '. . . he is a nice one . . . I could have killed him, I could kill him now.' There was a dreadful undertone in his voice as if he were ready to commit such a deed but also as if he would know that this would mean the destruction of all that he valued most.

Before he left he said: 'Since my wife and Peter have gone to the Clinic things are a little better at home. I stopped the television set as a punishment but now I have allowed it again.'

During the course of his treatment Peter frequently showed how deeply he suffered from his parents' quarrels. His relationships to both parents were good and he seemed to be a sort of mediator between them.

When he once said: 'Mummy and Daddy had another

row . . . I wish that they would love each other,' he was asked: 'Would you like to say a little prayer about this?'

He folded his hands and said: 'Dear God, I love Mummy and Daddy, I wish that they would love each other as Uncle Tom and Auntie Bessie do.'

During the mother's treatment she made bitter accusations against her husband and behaved aggressively towards the doctor. She was allowed to pour out her heart but then she was asked why she was so aggressive. This question evoked great emotion in her and she cried: 'Oh, I am not aggressive. I do care for my husband; if he needs me I shall stick to him. I love him.'

She was told that the happiness of her family depended on her abandoning her over-indulgence in her sons and in her love and loyalty for her husband and his beliefs.

The family situation showed some improvement, mother and father were talking to each other more than they did before, but it became increasingly clear that the most tragic conflict existed between the father and Robert and that no satisfactory solution could be found without improving this conflict. Indeed, Peter's difficulties appeared to be relatively less important than Robert's. An appointment with Robert at the Clinic was therefore arranged.

Robert was a well-mannered young man. He was depressed and apprehensive and one could see that he suffered severely. He related his terrible experience with his father: 'My father's face went livid . . . he was terrible . . . he looked as if he meant to kill me . . . we struggled . . . my mother came and separated us . . . my father was, perhaps, jealous . . . of course, I love my mother . . . I tried to approach him afterwards, but he would not climb down.'

Since he had been turned out of the house, Robert had found a girl whom he intended to marry. In the light of this his relationship to his mother was discussed with him and he showed insight into the danger of an unhealthy attachment to her. When he was asked if he wished to reconcile himself with his father, he affirmed this with sincerity. He was then asked if he was prepared to accept his father's nature and to try to sympathize with his father's feelings and outlook on life. Robert agreed to this.

When the father was told about Robert's wish to meet him he was furious and on the verge of an outburst. 'No! No! Everything is finished!' he said in despair. But there was an uncertainty in his voice and the date and place of the proposed meeting were made known to him.

The meeting between father and son was arranged not at the Clinic but at the more homely atmosphere of a private house. At the appointed time the father was the first to turn up. He wore his best suit and his face looked solemn and expectant. Robert arrived a little later, also in his best suit. He showed signs of fear and slightly trembled. They met quietly and did not talk much at first. But when the doctor left the room they began talking with each other in quiet, engaging voices. They had a long and good talk, lasting an hour, about home, the garden, Robert's work and intended marriage. When they went out into the road and their steps could be heard as they walked together, the text of Genesis appeared to be revived: '. . . so they went both of them together.'

The parts recorded of this case history are incomplete but they may serve as examples of how psychological phenomena can be interpreted in the light of the Akedah Motif. In interpreting Akedah experiences it ought to be born in mind that they should not be expected to correspond in detail to the pattern of the Biblical Akedah story. This story is a unique condensation of dramatic happenings in time, place and intensity. The Akedah experiences of everyday life usually develop slowly, inconspicuously, and incompletely. These everyday experiences show, however, the main features of the Akedah Motif: the struggle between two apparently equally good principles; the search for a solution; and phenomena which can best be interpreted by the assumption of the interference by an external moral power.

The father, when he came to the Clinic, was in a state of moral masochism. He was torn between two apparently good principles and could not find a redeeming solution. On the one hand his Laius Complex urged him to punish his family, an urge which was powerfully reinforced by his belief in law and order. This belief, obsessional as it was, was more than mere imitation of discipline learned in the Army. It was an expression of his belief in a super-natural order. On the other hand he was longing to show his tender love for his wife and sons, again as an expression of his love of God.

When the meeting with his son was offered to him his agony was at its height. Once more he behaved as if everything he valued was lost. But then a change took place in his mind and he came to the meeting, arriving there even before his son.

The mother, at the beginning of treatment, was still deeply involved in her Jocasta Complex. It was possible to resolve this complex to a large extent. She learned that, hidden under the rigid discipline of her husband, were valuable features and she began to influence her sons to value them too. In her love for her husband and sons she always was a mediator but it was not before she learned to give up her Jocasta Complex and to accept her husband's values that she became what can, symbolically, be called an angel-like figure in the struggle between father and sons.

Robert too was in a state of moral masochism when he was seen at the Clinic. He had the vision of submitting himself to his father, not only to his authority, but also to his values. He was helped in this by his mother and also by his fiancée and little brother. Peter, through his love, and in spite of his own difficulties, helped his father during the time of his greatest despair and prepared the way for his reconciliation with Robert.

The change of mind, or turning, of the persons of the drama was a process of gaining new insight. It was brought about not suddenly but by a long struggle of tender love with aggressive impulses. Adjustment to the reality situation with the assistance of explanations suggested during treatment was helpful but, in the last instance, the process was invoked by experiences which are best defined as religious experiences. They were derived from a belief in spiritual values and, in some aspects, strikingly resembled experiences as they are related in the Akedah story.

Conclusions

'And he shall turn the heart of the fathers to the children, and the heart of the children to their fathers.'

MALACHI, IV, 6

'For, behold, I create new heavens and a new earth.'

ISAIAH, LXV, 17

Conclusions

THE Akedah Motif is the Biblical aspect of the psychology of family relationships. It is the Biblical extension of the Oedipus Complex. The similarities and differences in the psycho-sexual approach of *the Oedipus Complex* and in the psycho-Biblical approach of *the Akedah Motif* will now be shortly reviewed.

The Oedipus Complex is the nuclear or central complex of normal psychological development and of all neurotic disturbances. The Akedah Motif, in a similar way, is the basic experience of Biblical religion, being, as it were, a prelude to the Decalogue, the Gospels and the Koran. The Akedah holds therefore, until this day, a central place in Jewish, Christian and Islamic beliefs.

The Oedipus Complex is conceived as a biological phenomenon which fits completely in the scheme of natural evolution. The Akedah Motif is a religious phenomenon which recognizes biological evolution but gives it Biblical meaning. It springs from the belief that human destiny is influenced by the external moral power of God.

The development of the Oedipus Complex follows the laws of gradual development of biology. According to the Biblical view, which is accepted in this study, the Akedah Motif, as the result of Divine intervention, developed suddenly in history, at a definite time and place and in definite ciscumstances. Before this historic event a gradual development of Akedah tendencies amongst all nations of the world prepared the way for the full Akedah experience.

The Oedipus Complex develops during the stages of psycho-sexual development of the child. The Akedah Motif has its beginning in childhood and develops fully in adulthood. Whilst in the Oedipus Complex the emphasis is on the experiences of the child, as the name of Oedipus Complex implies, the emphasis in the Akedah Motif is on the mutual experiences of parent and child. The initiative in this process is with the parent.

The resolution of the Oedipus Complex is brought about by the emergence of the super-ego. Its main sources are the introjection of parental and other images and secondary narcissism and its main effects are moralization, moral masochism and instinct transformation. The concept of super-ego formation is basic also for the Akedah Motif. But from the Biblical point of view the super-ego, as postulated by Freud, only describes the compromise solution of the Oedipus Complex. The Biblical, that is, the full solution of the problems of filio-parental relationships, requires an extended view of the present super-ego concept.

According to our interpretation of the Akedah Motif the image of man's divine calling is introjected, in addition to the images of the parents. The introjected call of God contains an altruistic aim and therefore love for this ego-ideal decreases narcissistic love and increases object-love. The moral masochism and the As If experience play a dominant role in the Akedah Motif. The torturing inner struggle is overcome by the choice to follow the altruistic call. This is the turning point in the Akedah experience. It is accompanied by a modification of instincts. The life instinct and desire for action are promoted, and the death instinct and contentment with meditation only are relegated. Object-love is amplified to embrace all human beings and future generations. It becomes messianic love.

Modern pysychology is to a great extent based on *non-Biblical ideas.* They are mainly of ancient Greek or Chinese or Indian origin.

The very word 'psyche' is Greek. The central psychoanalytic concept of the formation of character and neurosis is shaped after the Greek Oedipus myth. It is undoubtedly true that the great Greek thinkers possessed an understanding of the human mind which, in some respect, is unsurpassed to the present day and that the Trilogy of Sophocles still presents us with the most challenging problems. But stirring as these problems are they were not solved in the Tragedy of Oedipus. In ancient Greek philosophy only a heroic fight for the solution but no real solution is possible. Ancient Greek philosophy has not the vision of salvation.

In analytical psychology, Taoistic and Buddhistic elements provide leading ideas. But great as they are they teach self-centredness as the highest aim and fail in giving the redeeming solution of life.

No positive use has been made, so far, of the leading ideas of Biblical belief in the attempts of modern psychology to formulate basic findings and theories. But there is no reason why the *Bible* should not prove at least if not more fruitful than the concepts of Greek or Eastern religious experience.

Psychology and theology are at the cross-roads. The atheistic and pantheistic aspects of modern psychology lead to dangerous conclusions. The non-biological aspect of theology is doomed to lead to frustration. Psychology and theology must fructify each other, forming a synthetic science. Indian and Chinese religions have already contributed to the development of psychological systems. There is a need for a Biblical psychology.

Conclusions

Biblical psychology would accept the reality and the uniqueness of the God of Biblical religion.

It would have to recognize other personal Biblical experiences in addition to the Akedah experience.

In contrast to the phenomenon of self-realization of Eastern psychologies, the highest therapeutic aim of Biblical psychology would be the theme of messianic object-love.

It is the author's conviction that studies in Biblical psychology provide a necessary requirement for the development of psychiatry. It is hoped that further research along the lines indicated will contribute to this development.

Bibliography

ANTHROPOLOGY AND MYTHOLOGY

DE GROAT, J. J. M. (1901). *The Religious System of China*, Vol. II, Book I. *Disposal of the Dead*, Vol. IV, Book II. On the Soul and Ancestral Worship. (Leiden: E. J. Brill.)

EURIPIDES (1950). *Iphigenia in Aulis*. Done into English Verse by S. Claude Tickell. (London: University Research Society.)

FRANKFORT, H. (1951). 'The Problem of Similarity in Ancient Near Eastern Religions.' The Frazer Lecture, 1950. (Oxford: At the Clarendon Press.)

FRAZER, J. G. (1919). *Folk-Lore in the Old Testament*, Vol. I. (London: Macmillan.)

FRAZER, J. G. (1930). *The Golden Bough. A Study in Magic and Religion*, 3rd Edition, Part III, The Dying God. (London: Macmillan.)

MACCULLOCH, J. A. (1948). *The Celtic and Scandinavian Religions*. (London: Hutchinson's University Library.)

SMITH, R. BROUGH. (1878). *The Aborigines of Victoria*. (Melbourne and London.)

SPENCE, L. (1927). *The Myths of Mexico and Peru*. (London, Bombay, Sydney: George G. Harrap.)

STURLESON, SNORRE (1844). *The Heimskringla, or Chronicles of the Kings of Norway*. Vol. I. Translated from the Islandic by S. Laing. (London: Longman, Brown, Green and Longmans.)

THE OXFORD CLASSICAL DICTIONARY (1949). (Oxford: At the Clarendon Press.)

Bibliography

THE STANDARD DICTIONARY OF FOLKLORE, MYTHOLOGY AND LEGEND. Edited by Maria Leach (1950). Two Volumes. (New York: Funk & Wagnalls.)

PSYCHOLOGY AND PHILOSOPHY

ABRAHAM, K. (1949). *Selected Papers on Psycho-Analysis.* 4th Impression. Translated by Douglas Bryan and Alix Strachy. (London: Hogarth Press and the Institute of Psycho-Analysis.)

ADLER, A. (1945). *Social Interest: A Challenge to Mankind.* Translated by J. Linton and Richard Vaughan. 3rd Impression. (London: Faber & Faber.)

ADLER, G. (1948). *Studies in Analytical Psychology.* (London: Routledge and Kegan Paul Ltd.)

BAIN, R. N. (1905). *The First Romanovs.*

FERENCZI, S. (1926). *Further Contributions to the Theory and Technique of Psycho-Analysis.* Compiled by J. Rickman. Translated by Elizabeth Suttie. (London: Hogarth Press.)

FLUGEL, J. C. (1921). *The Psycho-Analytic Study of the Family.* (London: Hogarth Press.)

FREUD, ANNA (1947). In: *Child Health and Development.* Edited by R. W. E. Ellis. (London: J. & A. Churchill.)

FREUD, S. (1900). *The Interpretation of Dreams.* Authorized translation of 3rd Edition, with Introduction by A. A. Brill. (London: G. Allen and Unwin.)

FREUD, S. (1950). *Totem and Taboo*, revised edition. Translated by James Strachey. (London: Routledge and Kegan Paul Ltd.)

FREUD, S. (1927). *The Ego and the Id.* (London: Hogarth Press.)

FREUD, S. (1922). *Group Psychology and Analysis of the Ego.* (London: Hogarth Press.)

FREUD, S. (1949) *Three Essays on the Theory of Sexuality.* Translated by James Strachey. (London: Imago Publishing Company.)

FREUD, S. (1933). *New Introductory Lectures on Psychoanalysis.* Translated by W. J. H. Sprott. (London: Hogarth Press.)

FROMM, E. (1948. 'The Oedipus Complex and the Oedipus Myth.' In: *The Family: Its Function and Destiny*, Vol .V., The Science of

Culture Series, edited by Ruth Nanda Anshen. (New York: Harper & Brothers.)

FROMM, E. (1952). *The Forgotten Language. An Introduction to the Understanding of Dreams, Fairy Tales and Myths.* (London: V. Gollancz.)

GLOVER, E. (1949). *Psycho-Analysis.* Second Edition. (London: Staples Press.)

GOSSE, E. (1907). *Father and Son. A Study of Two Temperaments.* (London: Heinemann.)

HINSIE, L. E., and SCHATZKY, J. (1940). *Psychiatric Dictionary.* (Oxford University Press.)

HOUSMAN, A. E. (1916). *A Shropshire Lad.* (London: Grant Richards.)

JUNG, C. G. (1917). On Psycho-Analysis. (Paper given before the 17th International Medical Congress, London, 1913.) In: *Two Essays on Analytical Psychology.* Translated by R. F. C. Hull. (London: Routledge and Kegan Paul Ltd.) (1953)

JUNG, C. G. (1919). *Psychology of the Unconscious.* Authorized translation with Introduction by Beatrice M. Hinkle. (London: Kegan Paul, Trench, Trubner & Co.)

KIERKEGAARD, SÖREN (1939). *Fear and Trembling,* Translated by R. Payne. (Oxford University Press.)

MULLAHY, P. (1948). *Oedipus, Myth and Complex. A Review of Psycho-Analytical Theory.* Introduction by E. F. Fromm. (London: G. Allen & Unwin.)

PAULY (1916). *Real-Encyclopaedie der Classischen Altertumswissenschaft.* 9. Band. (Stuttgard: J. B. Metzler.)

PORPHYRY. *De Abstinentia.* (Paris: Ed. R. Hercher.) (1858)

RANK, O. (1926). *The Trauma of Birth.* (London: Kegan Paul, Trench, Trubner.)

ROBERT, C. (1915). *Oidipus, Geschichte eines poetischen Stoffs im Griechischen Altertum.* 2 Bände. (Berlin: Weidmannsche Buchhandlung.)

ROSCHER, W. H. (1897-1902). *Ausführliches Lexikon der Griechisches und Römischen Mythologie.* 3. Band. (Leipzig: Teubner.)

SOPHOCLES (1948). *Oedipus at Colonnus.* Translated into English rhyming Verse with Introduction and Notes by Gilbert Murray. (London: Allen & Unwin.)

SOPHOCLES (1947). *The Theban Plays.* A new translation by E. F. Watling. The Penguin Classics. (Harmondsworth Penguin Books Ltd.)

STERN, E. S. (1948). 'The Medea Complex: The Mother's Homicidal Wishes to her Child.' *Journ. of Mental Science*, Vol. XCIV, No. 395.

VAIHINGER, H. (1924). *The Philosophy of As If: A System of the Theoretical, Practical and Religious Fictions of Mankind.* (London: Kegan Paul.)

WALKER-PUNER, HELEN (1949). *Freud, his Life and his Mind. A Biography.* (London: The Grey Walls Press.)

THEOLOGY

Judaism

ASHER, D. (1866). *Selichoth. The Daily Morning Prayers.* (London: P. Vallentine.)

BEER, B. (1859). *Leben Abraham's nach Auffassung der jüdischen Sage. Mit erläuternden Anmerkungen und Nachweisungen.* (Leipzig: Oskar Leiner.)

DER MIDRASCH BERESCHIT RABBA. (Year of publication not stated.) Ins Deutsche ünertragen von A. Wuensche. (Leipzig: Otto Schultze.)

DUKES, L. (1842). *Zur Kenntnis der Neuhebräischen Religiösen Poesie.* (Frankfurt am Main: Bachsche Buchdruckerei.)

FRIEDLANDER, G. (1916). *Pirkê de Rabbi Eliezer. Rabbi Eliezer the Great.* (London: Kegan Paul, Trench, Trubner.)

GASTER, M. HAHAM (1928). *The Book of Prayer and Order of Service according to the Custom of the Spanish and Portuguese Jews.* English translation. Vol. II. *The Order of Service for the New Year.* (London: Oxford University Press.)

GINZBERG, L. (1909). *The Legends of the Jews.* Translated from the German Manuscript by Henriette Szold. Vol. I. *Bible Times and Characters from the Creation to Jacob.* (Philadelphia: The Jewish Publication Society of America.)

Bibliography

HERSHON, P. I. (1885). *A Rabbinical Commentary on Genesis.* Translated from the Judaeo-Polish with Notes and Indices. (London: Hodder & Stoughton.)

JACOB, B. (1934). *Das Erste Buch der Thora. Genesis.* (Berlin: Schocken Verlag.)

JOSEPHUS FLAVIUS (1852–53). *Antiquitates Judaicae. Jüdische Altertümer.* Two volumes. Translated into German by K. Martin. (Köln.)

MICHA JOSEF BIN GORION (1914). *Die Sagen der Juden. Die Erzväter.* (Frankfurt am Main: Rütten & Loenig.)

MIDRASCH RABBAH (1939). Translated into English with Notes, etc., under the Editorship of H. Freedman and M. Simon. Genesis, i. Vayera. (London: The Soncino Press.)

THE BABYLONIAN TALMUD (1938). Translated into English under the Editorship of I. Epstein. Abboth Rosh Hashana. (London: The Soncino Press.)

THE FESTIVAL PRAYERS according to the Ritual of the German and Polish Jews (1876). Vol. III. Additional Service for the Day of Atonement. (London: Ann Abrahams and Son.)

THE JEWISH ENCYCLOPEDIA (1925). Vol. I. (New York: Funk & Wagnalls.)

THE NEW AKEDAH. Sermon for the Week. November 3rd., 1944. (*The Jewish Chronicle.*)

ZUNZ. (1855). *Die Synagogale Poesie des Mittelalters.* (Berlin: Julius Springer.)

CHRISTIANITY

ATHANASIUS ST. (1844). *The Festal Epistles. A Library of Fathers of the Holy Catholic Church.* (Oxford: J. H. Parker & Co.)

CHEYNE, T. K. and J. SUTHERLAND (1914). *Encyclopaedia Biblica. A Dictionary of the Bible.* (London: Adam & Charles Black.)

CYRIL OF ALEXANDRIA ST. (1881). *A Library of Fathers of the Holy Catholic Church.* (Oxford and London: J. H. Parker & Co.)

DEANE, W. J. (1906). *Abraham: His Life and Time.* (London: James Nisbet & Co.)

Bibliography

DELITZSCH, F. (1894). *A New Commentary on Genesis*. Two volumes. (Edinburgh: T. & T. Clark.)

DILLMANN, A. (1897). *Genesis critically exegetically expounded.* Translated by W. B. Stevenson. In two volumes. (Edinburgh: T. & T. Clark.)

DODS, M. (1888). *The Book of Genesis. The Expositor's Bible.* (London: Hodder & Stoughton.)

DRIVER, S. R. (1906). *The Book of Genesis.* 5th Edition. *Westminster Commentaries.* Edited by W. Lock. (London: Methuen & Co.)

HASTINGS, J. (1900). *A Dictionary of the Bible.* (Edinburgh: T. & T. Clark.)

KAMPHAUSEN, D. A. (1896). *Das Verhältnis des Menschenopfers zur Israelitischen Religion.* (Bonn: Rörscheid & Ebbeke.)

MACLAREN, A. *The Book of Genesis. Exposition of Holy Scripture.* (London: Pickering & Inglis.)

LINNELL, J. (1844). *Burnt-Offering.* (London: E. Allen.)

QUANDT, E. (1871). *Maleachi,* der letzte Prophet des alten Bundes. (Berlin: Hauptverein für christliche Erbauungsschriften.)

RYLE, H. E. (1921). *The Book of Genesis. The Cambridge Bible.* (Cambridge University Press.)

SKINNER, J. (1912). *A Critical and Exegetical Commentary on Genesis. The International Critical Commentary.* (Edinburgh: T. & T. Clark.)

SPENCE, H. D. M. and J. S. EXELL (1897). *The Pulpit Commentary.* (London: Kegan Paul.)

THE CATHOLIC ENCYCLOPEDIA (1907). Vol. I. Edited by Ch. G. Herbemann. (New York: R. Appleton.)

THE HOLY BIBLE. *The Authorized Version.*

ISLAM

THE ENCYCLOPEDIA OF ISLAM (1927). Leyden: Late E. J. Brill. (London: Luzac & Co.)

THE KORAN. Translated into English from the original Arabic by G. Sale. (London: F. Warne & Co.)

WEILL (1846). *Biblical Legends of the Mussulmans.* (New York.)

Bibliography

ICONOGRAPHY

BODKIN, T. (1948). *Rembrandt, Paintings.* Apollo Edition. (London: Callius.)

LAW, E. (1927). *The New Authorised Historical Catalogue of the Pictures, Tapestries and Furniture in the King's Collection at Hampton Court.* (London: Hugh Rees.)

MARILLIER, H. C. (1951). *The Tapestries at Hampton Court Palace.* (London: Published for the Ministry of Works by Her Majesty's Stationery Office.)

SCHAPIRO, M. (1943). 'The Angel with the Ram in Abraham's Sacrifice: A Parallel in Western and Islamic Art. In: *Ars Islamica. The Research Seminar in Islamic Art.* (University of Michigan. Vol. X. Ann Arbor, University of Michigan Press.)

SMITH, A. M. (1922). 'The Iconography of the Sacrifice of Isaac in Early Christian Art. In: *American Journal of Archaeology.* Second Series. Vol. XXVI., No. 1. (The Rumford Press.)

THOMSON, W. G. (1930). *A History of Tapestry.* (London: Hodder & Stoughton.)

UNIVERSITY OF LONDON, THE WARBURG INSTITUTE (1949).

Author Index

Index

General Index

Index

Index

Index

Index

www.ingramcontent.com/pod-product-compliance
Lightning Source LLC
LaVergne TN
LVHW021111300926
849160LV00009B/691
* 9 7 8 0 4 1 5 8 6 5 4 7 0 *